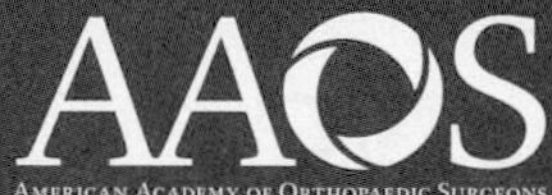

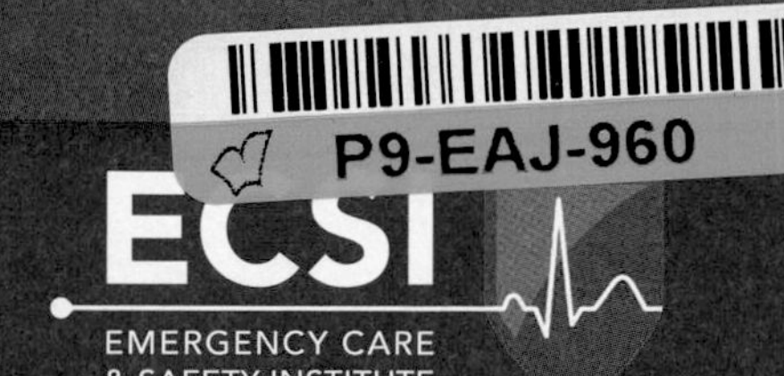

First Aid, CPR, and AED Standard

Seventh Edition

Alton L. Thygerson, EdD, FAWM
Medical Writer

Steven M. Thygerson, PhD, MSPH
Medical Writer

Benjamin Gulli, MD, FAAOS
Medical Editor

Howard L. Mell, MD, MPH, FACEP
Medical Editor

Bob Elling, MPA, EMT-P
Series Editor

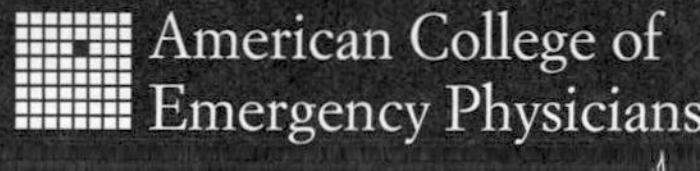

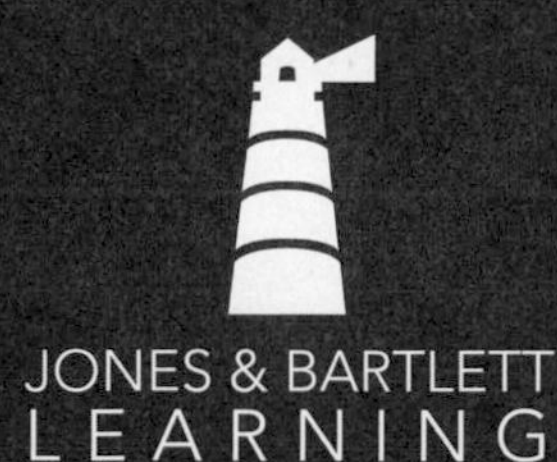

JONES & BARTLETT
LEARNING

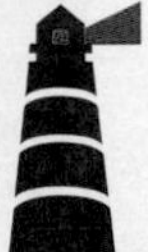

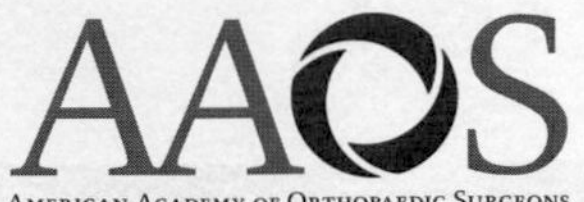

World Headquarters
Jones & Bartlett Learning
5 Wall Street
Burlington, MA 01803
978-443-5000
info@jblearning.com
www.jblearning.com

Editorial Credits
Chief Education Officer: Ellen C. Moore
Director, Department of Publications: Hans J. Koelsch, PhD
Managing Editor: Kimberly D. Hooker
Copy Editor: Jenna Skwarek

Jones & Bartlett Learning books and products are available through most bookstores and online booksellers. To contact Jones & Bartlett Learning directly, call 800-832-0034, fax 978-443-8000, or visit our website, www.jblearning.com.

Production Credits
General Manager, Executive Publisher: Kimberly Brophy
Director of Sales, Public Safety Group: Patricia Einstein
VP, Product Development and Executive Editor: Christine Emerton
Acquisitions Editor: Tiffany Sliter
Development Editor: Carly Mahoney
Senior Production Editor: Jessica deMartin
Marketing Manager: Jessica Carmichael
VP, Manufacturing and Inventory Control: Therese Connell
Composition: diacriTech
Cover Design: Kristin E. Parker
Rights & Media Specialist: Robert Boder
Media Development Editor: Troy Liston
Cover Image: © SeanShot/iStock/Getty; © Science Photo Library/Getty
Printing and Binding: RR Donnelley Kendallville

Library of Congress Cataloging-in-Publication Data
Names: Thygerson, Alton L., author. | Thygerson, Steven M., author. | American Academy of Orthopaedic Surgeons, issuing body. | American College of Emergency Physicians, issuing body.
Title: First aid, CPR, and AED. Standard / Alton L. Thygerson, Steven M. Thygerson; American Academy of Orthopaedic Surgeons, American College of Emergency Physicians.
Other titles: Standard first aid, CPR, and AED
Description: Seventh edition. | Burlington, MA : Jones & Bartlett Learning, [2017] | Includes index.
Identifiers: LCCN 2016004371 | ISBN 9781284041613
Subjects: | MESH: First Aid | Cardiopulmonary Resuscitation | Electric Countershock
Classification: LCC RC86.7 | NLM WA 292 | DDC 616.02/52—dc23
LC record available at http://lccn.loc.gov/2016004371

6048

Printed in the United States of America
20 19 18 17 16 10 9 8 7 6 5 4 3 2 1

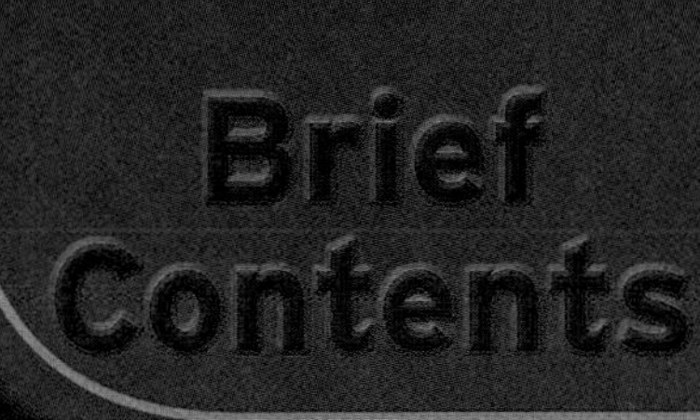
Brief
Contents

Contents

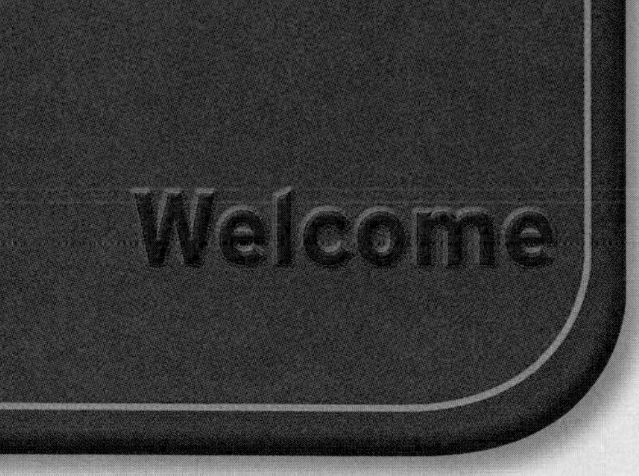

Welcome to the Emergency Care & Safety Institute

Welcome to the Emergency Care & Safety Institute (ECSI), brought to you by the American Academy of Orthopaedic Surgeons (AAOS) and the American College of Emergency Physicians (ACEP).

ECSI is an internationally renowned organization that provides training and certifications that meet job-related requirements as defined by regulatory authorities such as Occupational Safety & Health Administration (OSHA), The Joint Commission, and state offices of Emergency Medical Services (EMS), Education, Transportation, and Health. Our courses are delivered throughout a range of industries and markets worldwide, including colleges and universities, business and industry, government, public safety agencies, hospitals, private training companies, and secondary school systems.

ECSI programs are offered in association with the AAOS and ACEP. AAOS, the world's largest medical association of musculoskeletal specialists, is known as the original name in EMS publishing with the very first EMS textbook in 1971, and ACEP is widely recognized as the leading name in all of emergency medicine.

ECSI Course Catalog

Individuals seeking training from ECSI can choose from among various traditional classroom-based courses or alternative online courses such as:

- Automated External Defibrillation (AED)
- Bloodborne and Airborne Pathogens
- Babysitter Safety
- Driver Safety
- CPR (layperson and health care provider levels)
- First Aid (multiple courses available)
- Emergency Medical Responder
- Wilderness First Aid, and more!

ECSI offers a wide range of textbooks, instructor and student support materials, and interactive technology, including online courses. ECSI student manuals are the center of an integrated teaching and learning system that offers resources to better support instructors and train students. The instructor supplements provide practical hands-on, time-saving tools like PowerPoint presentations, DVDs, and web-based distance learning resources. Technology resources provide interactive exercises and simulations to help students become prepared for any emergency.

Documents attesting to ECSI's recognitions of satisfactory course completion will be issued to those who successfully meet the course requirements. Written acknowledgement of a participant's successful course completion is provided in the form of a Course Completion Card, issued by the Emergency Care & Safety Institute.

Visit www.ECSInstitute.org today!

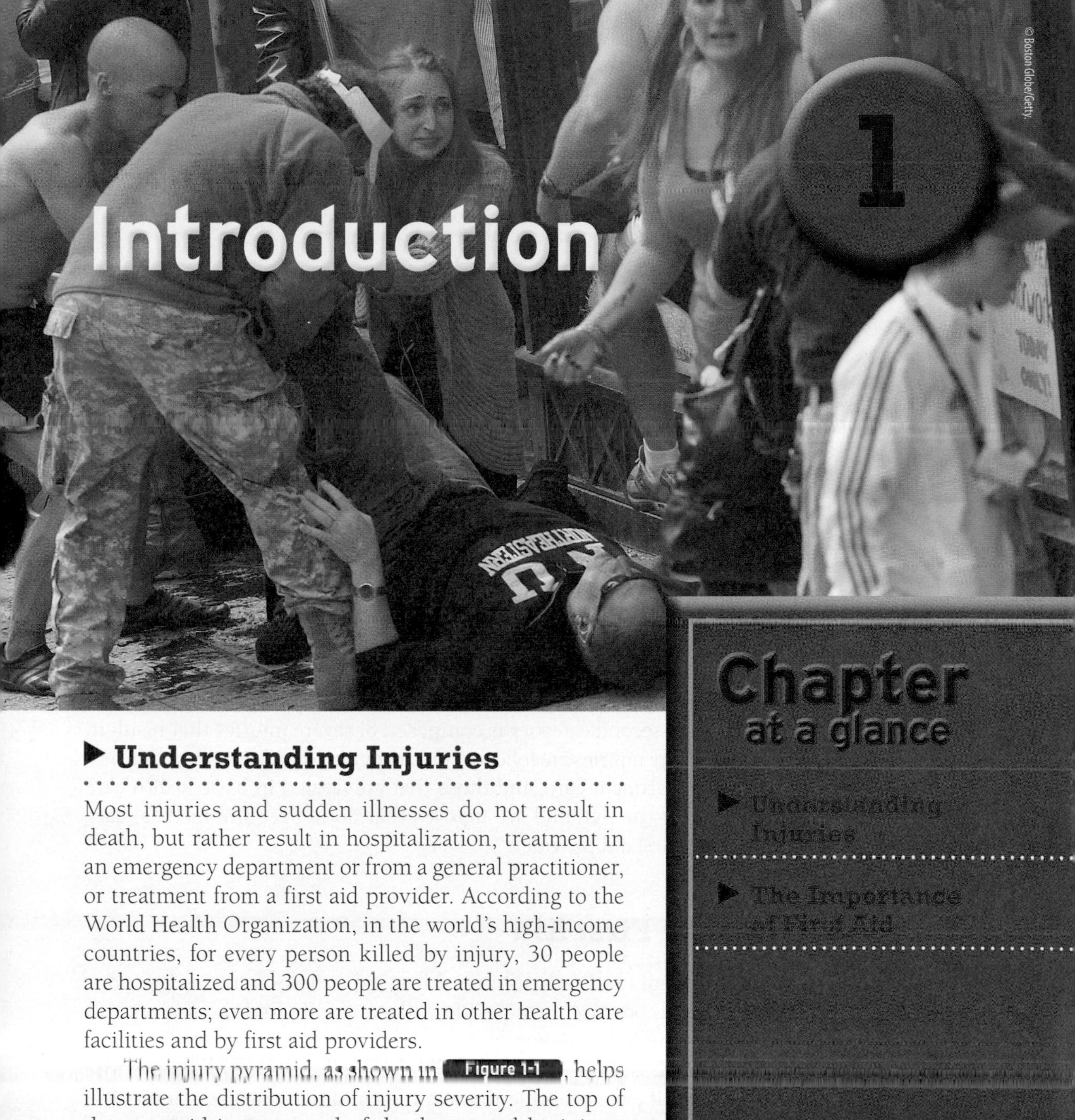

1 Introduction

Chapter at a glance

▶ Understanding Injuries

Most injuries and sudden illnesses do not result in death, but rather result in hospitalization, treatment in an emergency department or from a general practitioner, or treatment from a first aid provider. According to the World Health Organization, in the world's high-income countries, for every person killed by injury, 30 people are hospitalized and 300 people are treated in emergency departments; even more are treated in other health care facilities and by first aid providers.

The injury pyramid, as shown in Figure 1-1, helps illustrate the distribution of injury severity. The top of the pyramid is composed of deaths caused by injury. Although deaths from injury are fewer in number than other types of injuries, they are more visible because they are considered newsworthy and often appear on

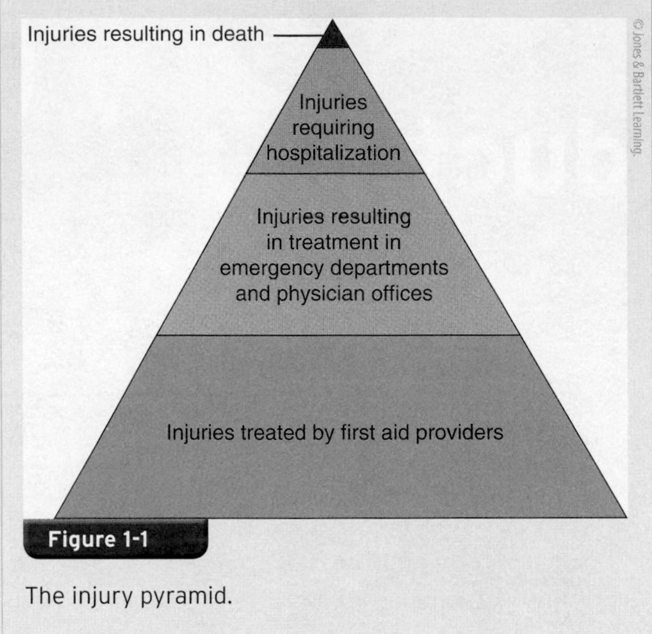

Figure 1-1

The injury pyramid.

television and in newspapers. The second category is composed of severe injuries that result in hospitalization and disability. Severe injuries are followed on the pyramid by less-severe injuries, those that require emergency department care, and those that are treated in basic health care facilities. Finally, at the bottom of the pyramid are injuries that do not require medical care and that are instead treated by a first aid provider.

▶ The Importance of First Aid

It is better to know first aid and not need it than to need first aid and not know it. Everyone should be able to provide first aid, because most people will eventually find themselves in a situation requiring it for another person or themselves.

Most injuries and sudden illnesses do not require lifesaving efforts. During their entire lifetimes, most people will rarely, if ever, see a life-threatening condition outside of a medical facility. Saving lives is important, but first aid providers are more frequently called upon to provide initial care for less-severe conditions. If not properly treated, these less-severe injuries can evolve into something more serious. As such, these skills demand attention during first aid training. The role of the first aid provider is discussed in **Flowchart 1-1**.

The latest International Liaison Committee on Resuscitation (ILCOR) guidelines define first aid as the helping behaviors and initial care provided for an acute illness or injury. According to the guidelines, the goals of the first aid provider include "preserving life, alleviating suffering, preventing further illness or injury, and promoting recovery." First aid, which

Flowchart 1-1 Role of the First Aid Provider

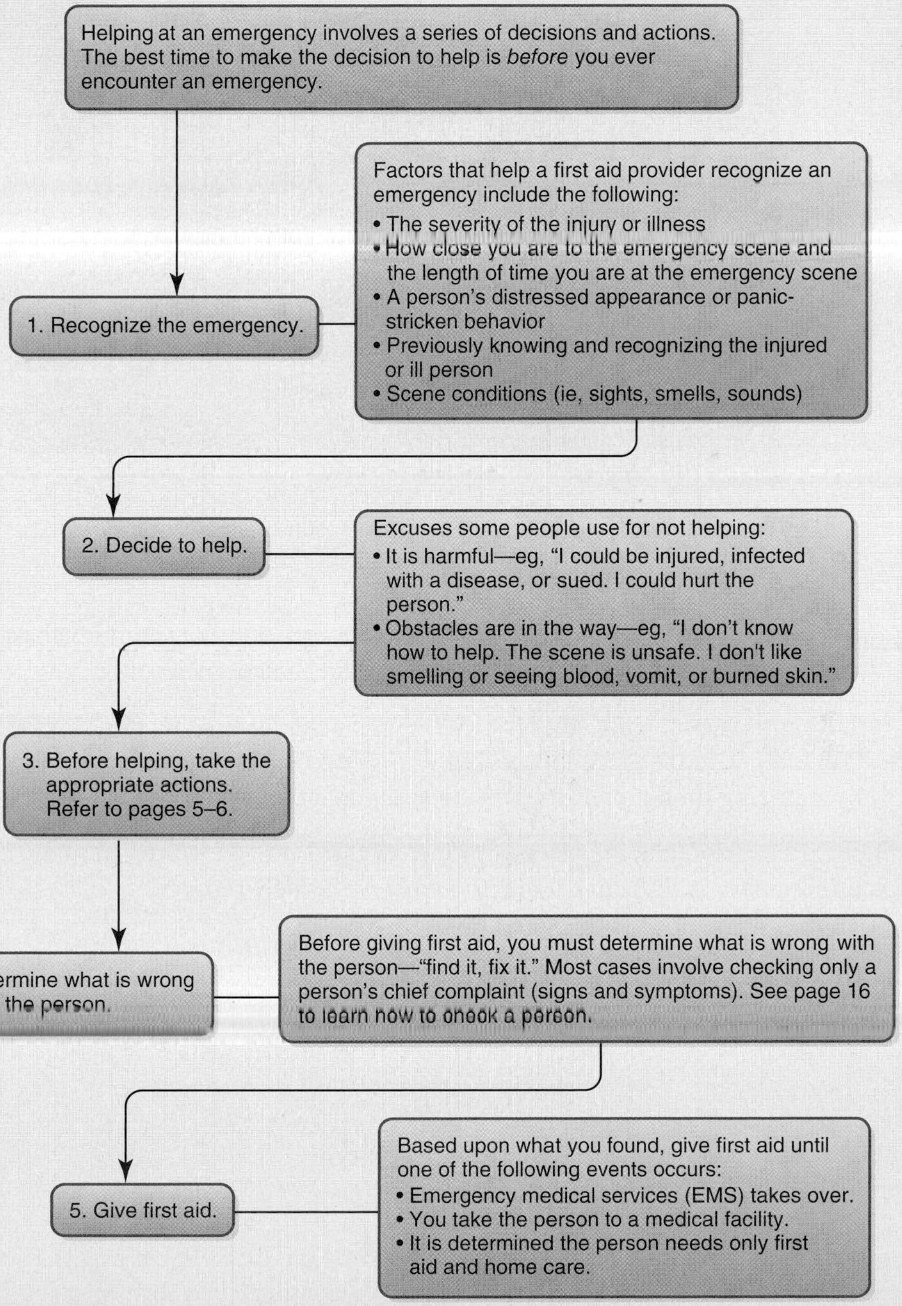

Helping at an emergency involves a series of decisions and actions. The best time to make the decision to help is *before* you ever encounter an emergency.

1. Recognize the emergency.

Factors that help a first aid provider recognize an emergency include the following:

- The severity of the injury or illness
- How close you are to the emergency scene and the length of time you are at the emergency scene
- A person's distressed appearance or panic-stricken behavior
- Previously knowing and recognizing the injured or ill person
- Scene conditions (ie, sights, smells, sounds)

2. Decide to help.

Excuses some people use for not helping:

- It is harmful—eg, "I could be injured, infected with a disease, or sued. I could hurt the person."
- Obstacles are in the way—eg, "I don't know how to help. The scene is unsafe. I don't like smelling or seeing blood, vomit, or burned skin."

3. Before helping, take the appropriate actions. Refer to pages 5–6.

4. Determine what is wrong with the person.

Before giving first aid, you must determine what is wrong with the person—"find it, fix it." Most cases involve checking only a person's chief complaint (signs and symptoms). See page 16 to learn how to check a person.

5. Give first aid.

Based upon what you found, give first aid until one of the following events occurs:

- Emergency medical services (EMS) takes over.
- You take the person to a medical facility.
- It is determined the person needs only first aid and home care.

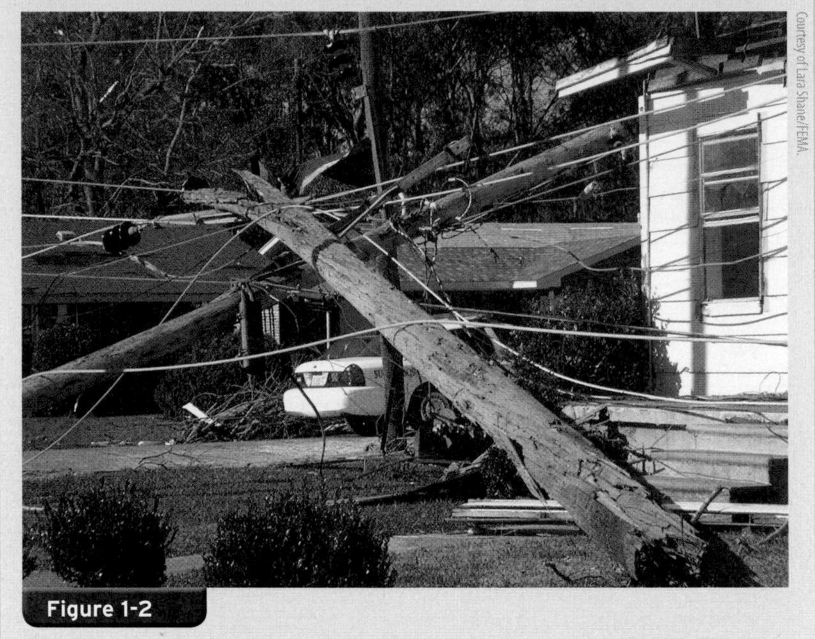
Courtesy of Lara Shane/FEMA.

Figure 1-2

The first step in providing first aid is to recognize an emergency exists.

includes self-care, can be initiated by anyone in any situation but should be based on medical and scientific evidence or expert consensus. First aid competencies include:

- Recognizing, assessing, and prioritizing the need for first aid Figure 1-2
- Providing care by using appropriate knowledge, skills, and behaviors
- Recognizing limitations and seeking additional care when needed

First aid does not take the place of proper medical care. However, in many cases, medical care is unnecessary and the ill or injured person will safely recover.

Before Helping, Take the Appropriate Actions

2

Chapter at a glance

▶ Introduction

This may be one of the most important sections in this manual. You must consider the actions in this section before helping an injured or suddenly ill person.

You have recognized an emergency and have decided to help. See page 3.

1. *Size up the scene.* See page 8.
   - Are dangerous hazards present?
   - How many people are involved? For multiple people, see pages 121–122.
   - What happened?
   - What is your first impression about what could be wrong with the person?
   - Are bystanders available to help?
2. *Ask if you may help.* If the person agrees, give first aid. If your help is refused and the injury or illness is serious, call 9-1-1. If the person is unresponsive, you can legally assume he or she

would accept your help. For a child, obtain the permission of a parent or legal guardian before giving first aid. If a parent or legal guardian is not present, you can legally assume that you have this person's permission to help his or her child. See pages 10–11.

3. *Seek medical care, if it is needed.* Depending upon the seriousness of the injury or illness and circumstances, either call 9-1-1 for emergency medical services (EMS) or take the person to a medical facility. If you are in a commercial building, then another option is to contact the company's emergency response team or security staff. You may decide to seek medical care immediately upon encountering a person with a severe condition or after you have determined what is wrong and provided first aid for the person. See pages 9–10.
4. *Prevent disease transmission.* Avoid contact with blood and other body fluids by putting on personal protective equipment (PPE). Disposable gloves, which are usually found in first aid kits, are the most commonly used type of PPE **Skill Sheet 2-1**. Less commonly used or available PPE include cardiopulmonary resuscitation (CPR) breathing masks with a one-way valve, and eye protection such as goggles or face shields that protect against spraying or splashing of blood or other body fluids. Handwashing is also effective in preventing disease transmission. See pages 11–13.

Note: Be aware that every situation is different. Depending on your relationship with the person (eg, spouse, parent), you may not need to wear PPE if you know his or her health history.

Skill Sheet

2-1 Removing Gloves

Note: **DO NOT** touch the outside of either glove with your bare hand.

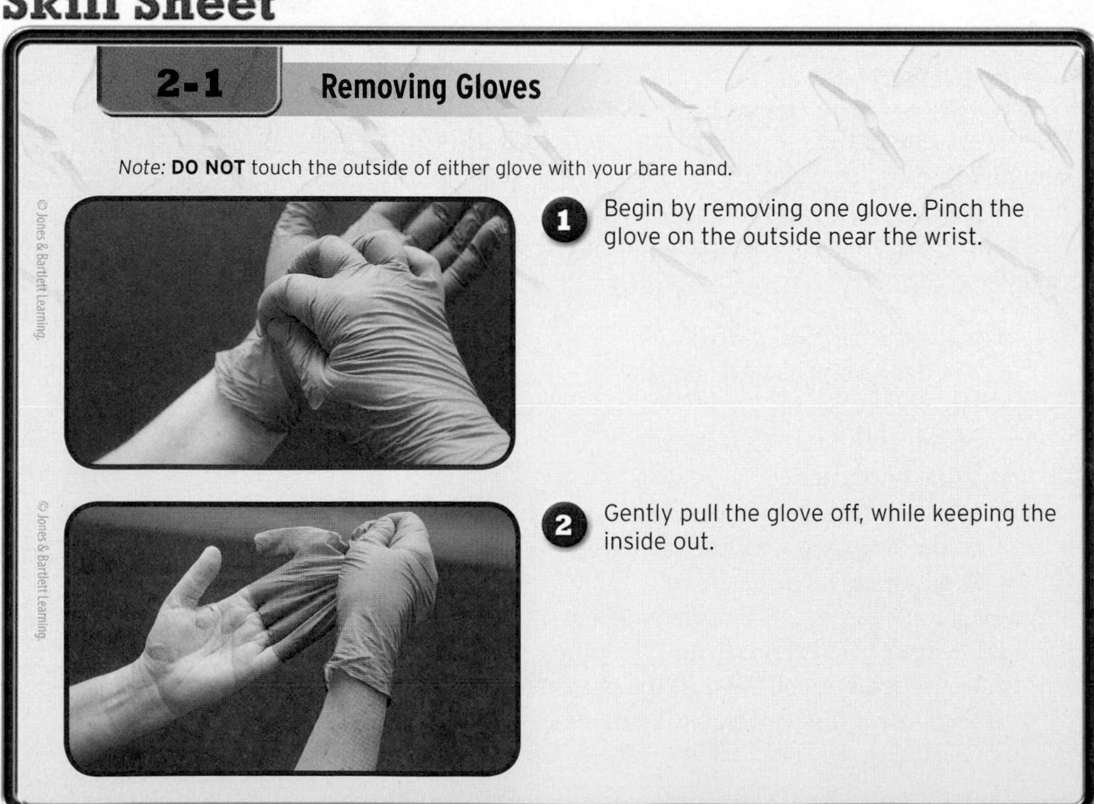

1. Begin by removing one glove. Pinch the glove on the outside near the wrist.

2. Gently pull the glove off, while keeping the inside out.

Skill Sheet Continued

2-1 Removing Gloves

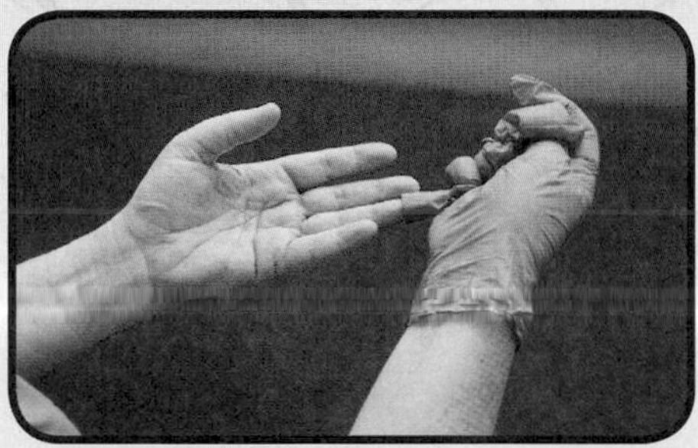

3 When removed, hold it in your gloved hand.

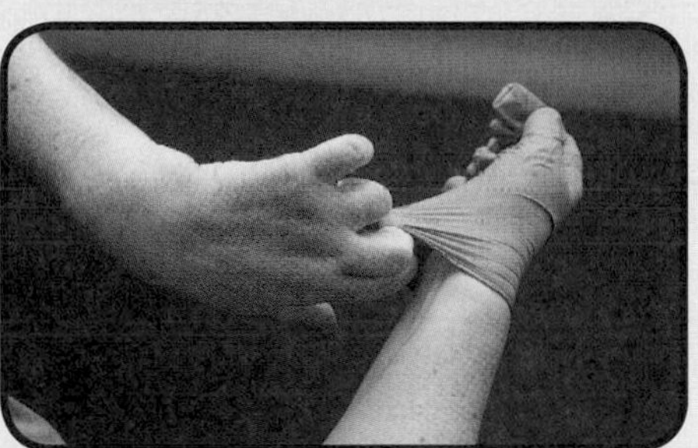

4 To remove the second glove, slide two fingers of your bare hand inside the remaining glove at the wrist.

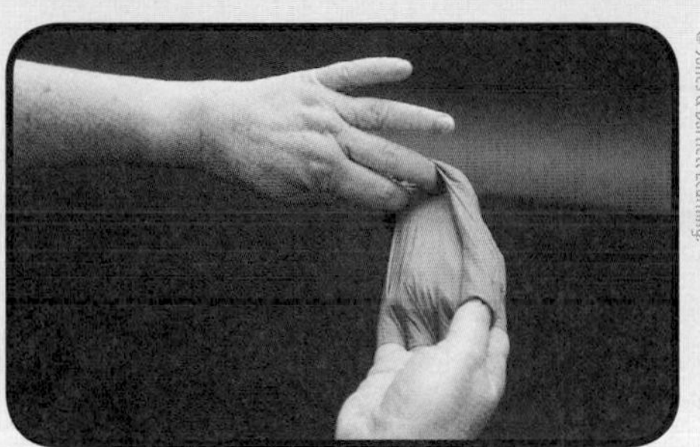

5 Gently stretch the glove away from the hand and gently pull the glove off, keeping the inside out. The first glove remains inside the second glove.

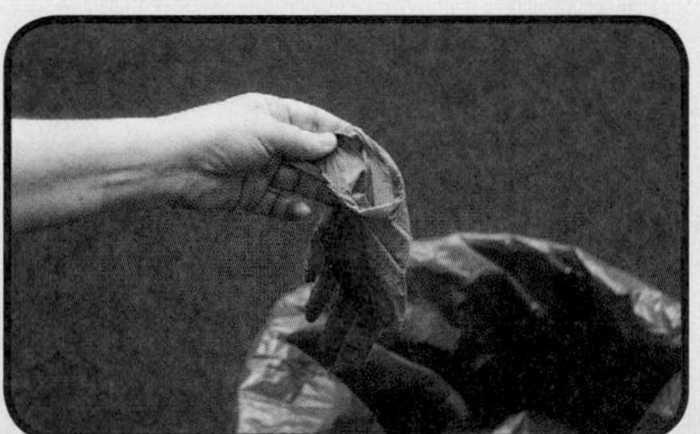

6 Dispose of the gloves in a biohazard container or a sealed plastic bag. Wash your hands with soap and running water. If they are not available, use an alcohol-based hand sanitizer.

Scene Size-up

You should perform a scene size-up every time you respond to an emergency. As you approach the scene, ask yourself a series of questions Flowchart 2-1.

Flowchart 2-1 Scene Size-up

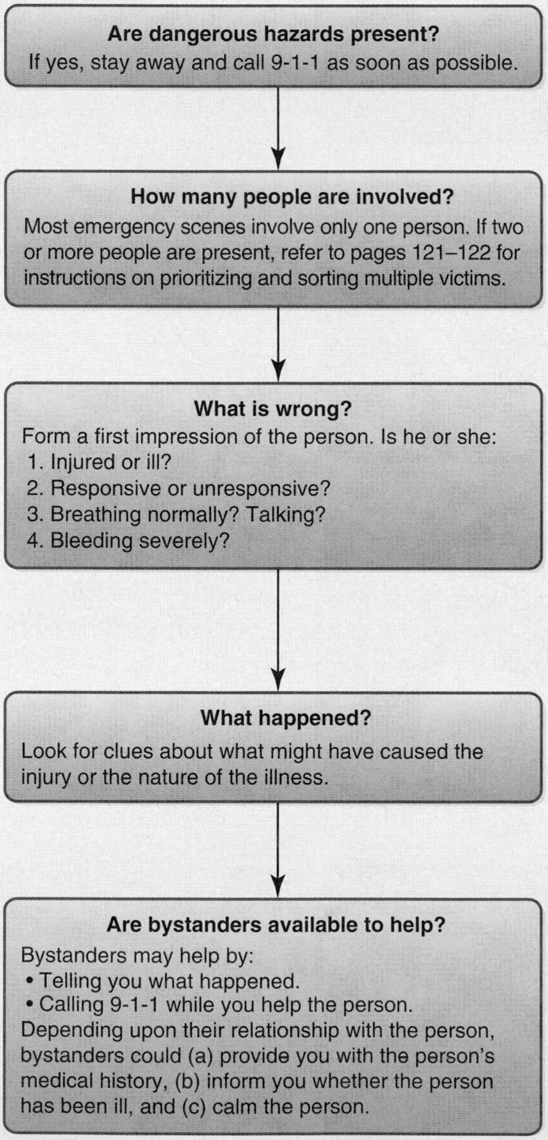

Are dangerous hazards present?
If yes, stay away and call 9-1-1 as soon as possible.

↓

How many people are involved?
Most emergency scenes involve only one person. If two or more people are present, refer to pages 121–122 for instructions on prioritizing and sorting multiple victims.

↓

What is wrong?
Form a first impression of the person. Is he or she:

1. Injured or ill?
2. Responsive or unresponsive?
3. Breathing normally? Talking?
4. Bleeding severely?

↓

What happened?
Look for clues about what might have caused the injury or the nature of the illness.

↓

Are bystanders available to help?
Bystanders may help by:

- Telling you what happened.
- Calling 9-1-1 while you help the person.

Depending upon their relationship with the person, bystanders could (a) provide you with the person's medical history, (b) inform you whether the person has been ill, and (c) calm the person.

Seeking Medical Care

You should recognize when medical care is needed and know how to get it. This includes learning how and when to access EMS by calling 9-1-1, how to activate the on-site emergency response system, and how to contact the Poison Control Center (1-800-222-1222) Figure 2-1.

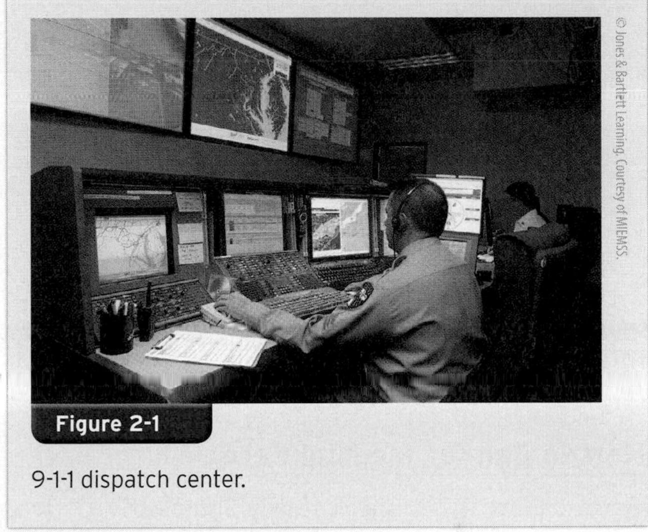

Figure 2-1

9-1-1 dispatch center.

When to Call 9-1-1

Not every cut requires stitches, nor does every burn require medical care. You may be confronted with the dilemma of whether to drive the person to the hospital or to call 9-1-1. According to the American College of Emergency Physicians (ACEP), you should call 9-1-1 for help if you answer "yes" to any of the following questions:

- Is the condition life-threatening?
- Could the condition get worse on the way to the hospital?
- If you move the person, will it cause further injury?
- Does the person need the skills or equipment of EMS?
- Would distance or traffic cause a delay in getting the person to the hospital?

If unsure about the answer to the above questions, call 9-1-1 and the trained dispatcher will advise you. It is better to be safe and call 9-1-1 when in doubt.

ACEP also recommends the immediate transport of people with the following conditions:

- Difficulty breathing, especially if it does not improve with rest
- Chest or upper abdominal pain or pressure lasting 2 minutes or more
- A fast heartbeat (more than 120 to 150 beats per minute) at rest, especially if associated with shortness of breath or feeling faint
- Fainting (passing out) or unresponsiveness
- Difficulty speaking, or numbness or weakness of any part of the body
- Sudden dizziness
- Confusion or changes in mental status, unusual behavior, or difficulty walking
- Sudden blindness or vision changes
- Bleeding from any wound that will not stop with direct pressure
- Broken bones visible through an open wound, or a broken leg
- Drowning
- Choking

- Severe burn
- Allergic reaction, especially if there is any difficulty breathing
- Extremely hot or cold body temperature
- Poisoning or drug overdose
- Sudden, severe headache
- Any sudden or severe pain
- Severe or persistent vomiting or diarrhea
- Coughing or vomiting of blood
- Behavioral emergencies (threatening to hurt or kill themselves or someone else)

Of course, this list does not represent every sign or symptom that might indicate a medical emergency. When unsure, call 9-1-1.

How to Call for Medical Care

When calling 9-1-1, speak slowly and clearly. Be ready to give the dispatcher the following information:

- The person's location
- The phone number you are calling from and your name
- A brief account of what happened
- The number of people needing help and any special conditions at the scene
- A description of the person's condition and what is being done

Listen to what the dispatcher tells you to do. If necessary, write down the instructions. Do not hang up until the dispatcher tells you to do so. Stay with the person needing help until EMS arrives.

9-1-1 Service

According to the National Emergency Number Association, over 98% of the people in the United States and Canada are covered by some type of 9-1-1 service. Many areas also have Enhanced 9-1-1, which allows the dispatcher to see the caller's phone number and address if the call is placed on a landline. When you call 9-1-1 from a cell phone, however, Enhanced 9-1-1 cannot identify your exact address, because cell phone signals only provide a general location. Because of this key difference, make sure you know your exact address or location to give the 9-1-1 dispatcher.

▶ Legal Aspects of First Aid

You may not be legally required to help another injured or ill person, but most people believe helping others is a moral obligation. You must help when you have a legal duty to act **Figure 2-2**:

- Employment requires it (ie, job description)
- Preexisting relationship exists (ie, parent-child, teacher-student, driver-passenger)

Good Samaritan laws provide reasonable protection against lawsuits and encourage people to assist others during an emergency. Laws vary from state to state but in general, the following conditions must be met:

- You are acting with good intentions.
- You are providing care without expectation of compensation.
- You are acting within the scope of your training.
- You are not acting in a grossly negligent (reckless) manner.

Negligent actions include:

- Giving substandard care
- Withholding care when you have a legal duty to act
- Causing injury or harm
- Exceeding your level of training
- Abandoning the person (starting care and then stopping or leaving without ensuring that a rescuer with the same or a higher level of training will continue to care for the person)

Always obtain consent (permission) before giving first aid. Types of consent include:

- Informed: Tell the person that you are trained and what you will be doing, and ask if you can help.
- Implied: Assume consent for an unresponsive or incompetent person.
- For children: Consent must be obtained from a parent or legal guardian unless unavailable, then implied consent can be assumed.

▶ Preventing Disease Transmission

Body fluids (such as blood, saliva, and stool) can sometimes carry disease-producing germs. Take standard precautions (also known as universal precautions or body substance isolation) Flowchart 2-2 to protect against diseases such as:

- AIDS/HIV
- Hepatitis B virus
- Hepatitis C virus
- Tuberculosis
- Meningitis

Avoid contact with blood and other body fluids by putting on PPE. PPE includes:

- Disposable gloves made of latex, nitrile, or vinyl (Use latex-free gloves if possible because some people are allergic to latex.) Figure 2-3
- Eye protection (goggles)
- Mouth-to-barrier device (face mask) when giving CPR Figure 2-4

Flowchart 2-2 Disease Prevention

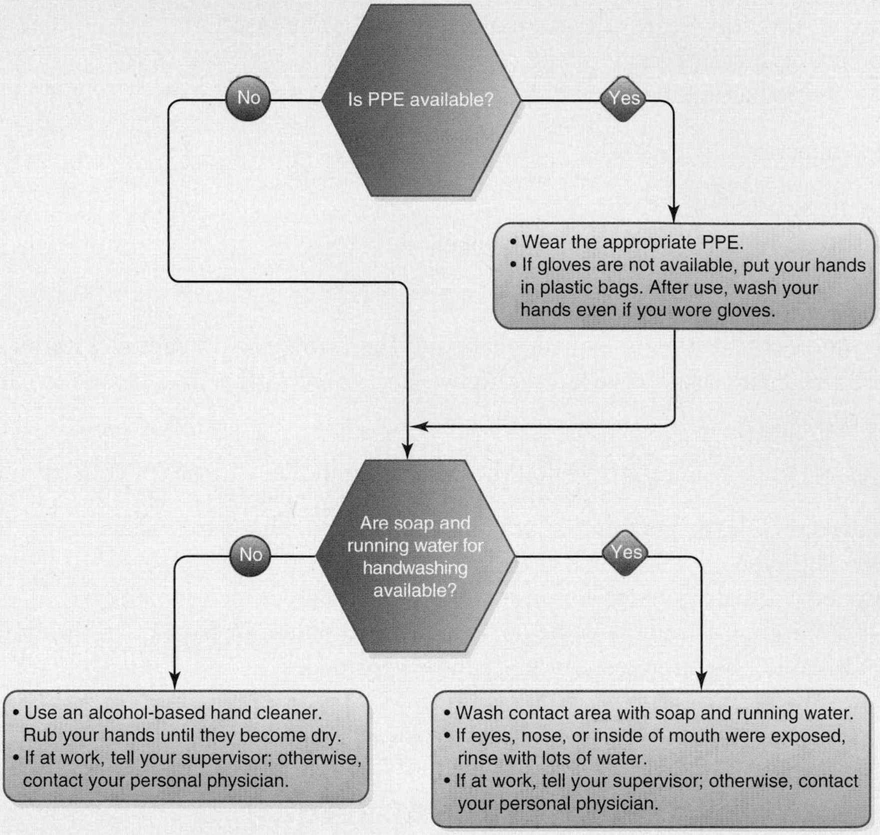

Is PPE available?

Yes:
- Wear the appropriate PPE.
- If gloves are not available, put your hands in plastic bags. After use, wash your hands even if you wore gloves.

No: proceed to next question.

Are soap and running water for handwashing available?

No:
- Use an alcohol-based hand cleaner. Rub your hands until they become dry.
- If at work, tell your supervisor; otherwise, contact your personal physician.

Yes:
- Wash contact area with soap and running water.
- If eyes, nose, or inside of mouth were exposed, rinse with lots of water.
- If at work, tell your supervisor; otherwise, contact your personal physician.

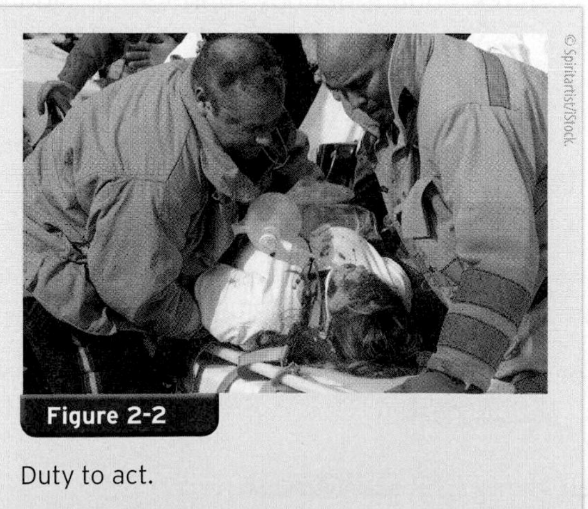

Figure 2-2

Duty to act.

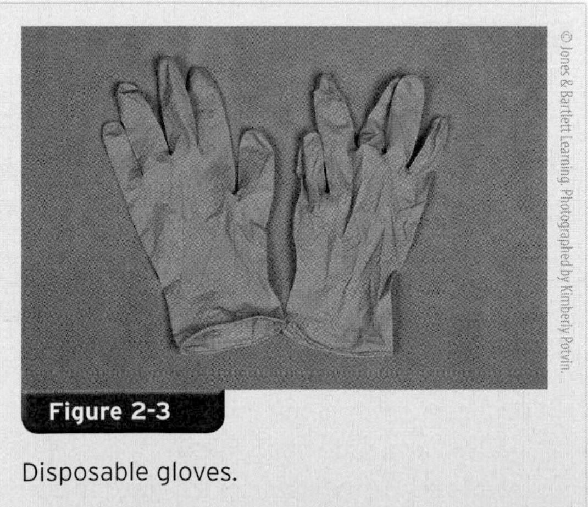

Figure 2-3

Disposable gloves.

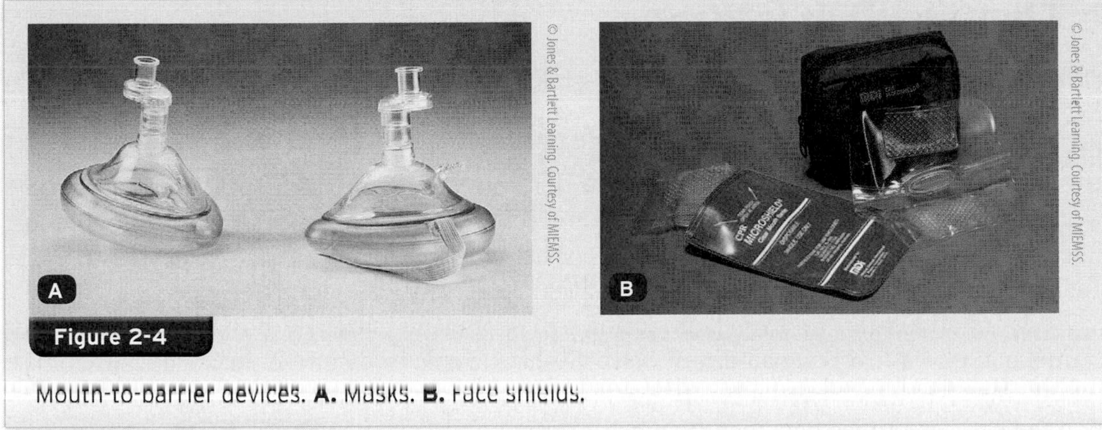

Figure 2-4

Mouth-to-barrier devices. **A.** Masks. **B.** Face shields.

Cleaning a Blood Spill

1. Wear PPE.
2. Wipe up blood with paper towels.
3. Spray or wash the area with 1 part liquid bleach in 9 parts water and let it air dry.
4. Dispose of materials in a biohazard container. If one is not available, double-bag in plastic bags.
5. When finished, wash your hands.

How to Wash Your Hands

Wash your hands as follows, if possible, before and after giving first aid (even if gloves were worn) **Figure 2-5**:

1. Wash your hands with soap and running water (use warm water when available).
2. Rub all hand surfaces together for 15 to 20 seconds.
3. Rinse off the soap with running water.
4. Dry your hands with a clean towel or a paper towel.

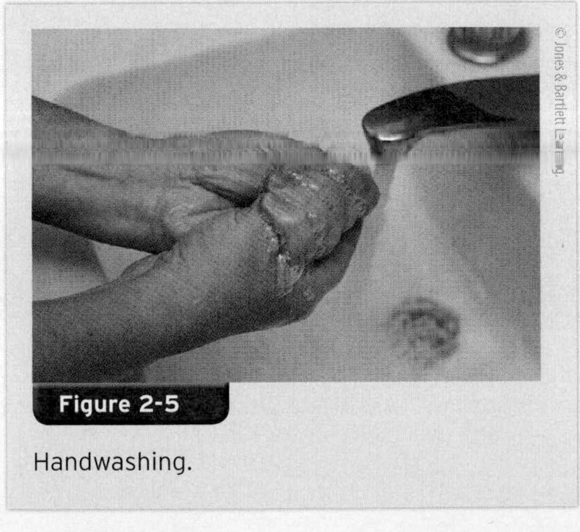

Figure 2-5

Handwashing.

▶ Finding What is Wrong

During emergency situations, it is crucial that you know what to do and what not to do **Flowchart 2-3**. Finding what is wrong helps reduce panic and ensure that safe and appropriate first aid is provided **Skill Sheet 2-2**.

The saying "Find it, fix it" stresses the idea that you cannot provide first aid unless you know what is wrong. Most ill or injured people do not require a complete assessment; you will most likely only need to ask the person about his or her chief complaint **Figure 2-6**. This process enables you to act quickly and decisively in hectic emergency situations.

If you find a significant problem during the assessment, stop and provide treatment. For a chief complaint involving an illness, you will not be able to diagnose the exact cause of the illness. Instead, determine if it is serious enough to require medical care. A medical identification tag can sometimes help identify what is wrong with a person **Figure 2-7**. If the person requires medical care, pass along the information you find during the assessment to the EMS personnel or health care providers.

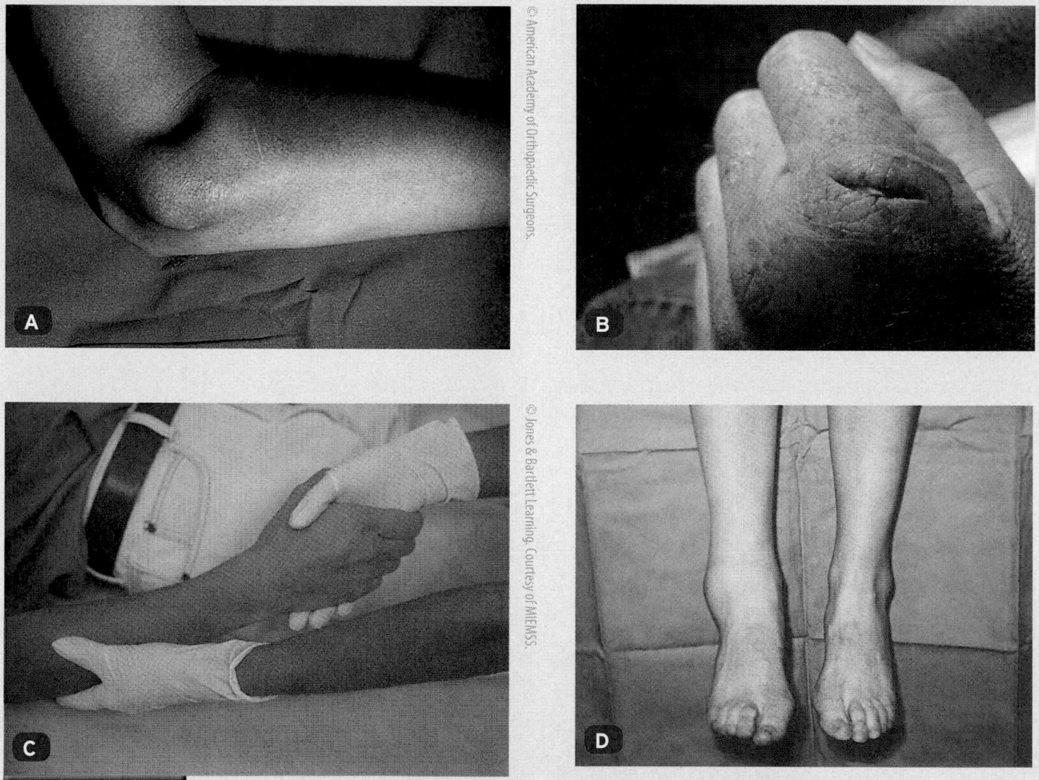

A

B

C

D

Figure 2-6

Check the person head to toe, looking, asking and feeling for DOTS: Deformities **(A)**, Open wounds **(B)**, Tenderness (pain) **(C)**, and Swelling **(D)**.

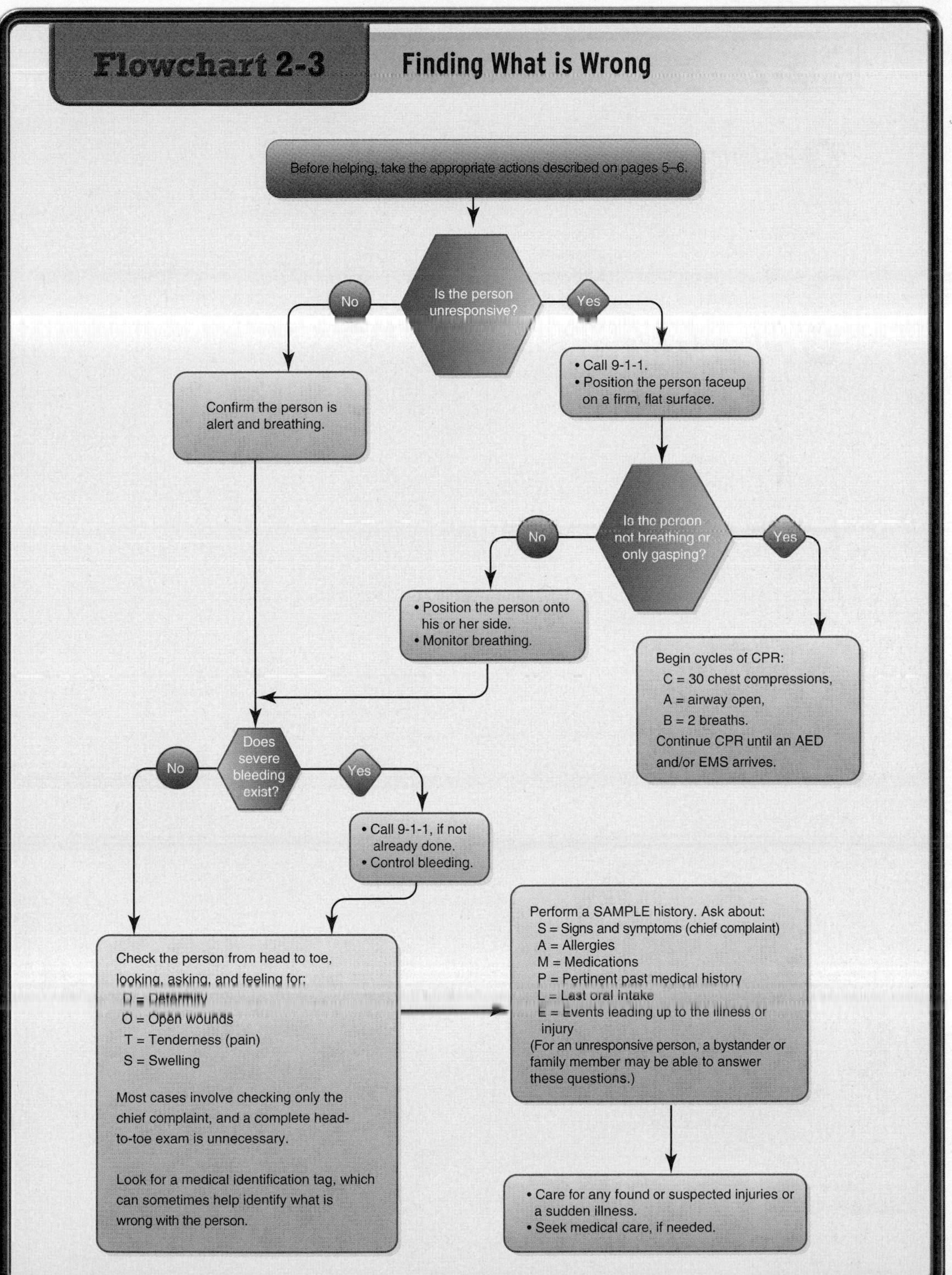
Flowchart 2-3
Finding What is Wrong
Before helping, take the appropriate actions described on pages 5–6.
Is the person unresponsive?
No
Yes
• Call 9-1-1.
• Position the person faceup on a firm, flat surface.
Confirm the person is alert and breathing.
Is the person not breathing or only gasping?
No
Yes
• Position the person onto his or her side.
• Monitor breathing.
Begin cycles of CPR:
C = 30 chest compressions,
A = airway open,
B = 2 breaths.
Continue CPR until an AED and/or EMS arrives.
Does severe bleeding exist?
No
Yes
• Call 9-1-1, if not already done.
• Control bleeding.
Check the person from head to toe, looking, asking, and feeling for:
D = Deformity
O = Open wounds
T = Tenderness (pain)
S = Swelling
Most cases involve checking only the chief complaint, and a complete head-to-toe exam is unnecessary.
Look for a medical identification tag, which can sometimes help identify what is wrong with the person.
Perform a SAMPLE history. Ask about:
S = Signs and symptoms (chief complaint)
A = Allergies
M = Medications
P = Pertinent past medical history
L = Last oral intake
E = Events leading up to the illness or injury
(For an unresponsive person, a bystander or family member may be able to answer these questions.)
• Care for any found or suspected injuries or a sudden illness.
• Seek medical care, if needed.

Skill Sheet

2-2 Finding What is Wrong with an Alert and Responsive Person

1 *Perform a primary assessment.*

Make eye contact, introduce yourself, and ask if you can help.

- Ask "What happened?" and "Where do you hurt?"
- Scan the body for any severe bleeding; if found, control it.
- If the person is severely injured, call 9-1-1 or ask another bystander to call.

Have the person move to a comfortable position (lying down or leaning against a stable object).

2 *Perform a secondary assessment.*

Physical Exam

Check the person from head to toe while looking, asking, and feeling for DOTS:

- D = Deformities
- O = Open wounds
- T = Tenderness (pain)
- S = Swelling

Look for a medical identification necklace or bracelet.

SAMPLE History

Use the SAMPLE mnemonic to help you identify what could be wrong. Ask about:

- S = Signs and symptoms (chief complaint)
- A = Allergies
- M = Medications
- P = Pertinent past medical history
- L = Last oral intake
- E = Events leading up to the illness or injury

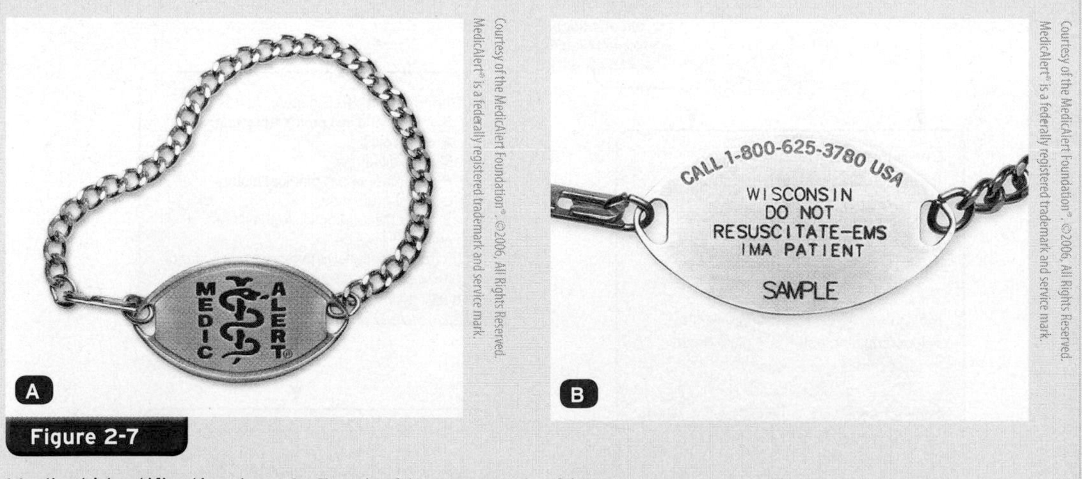

Figure 2-7

Medical identification tag. **A.** Front of tag. **B.** Back of tag.

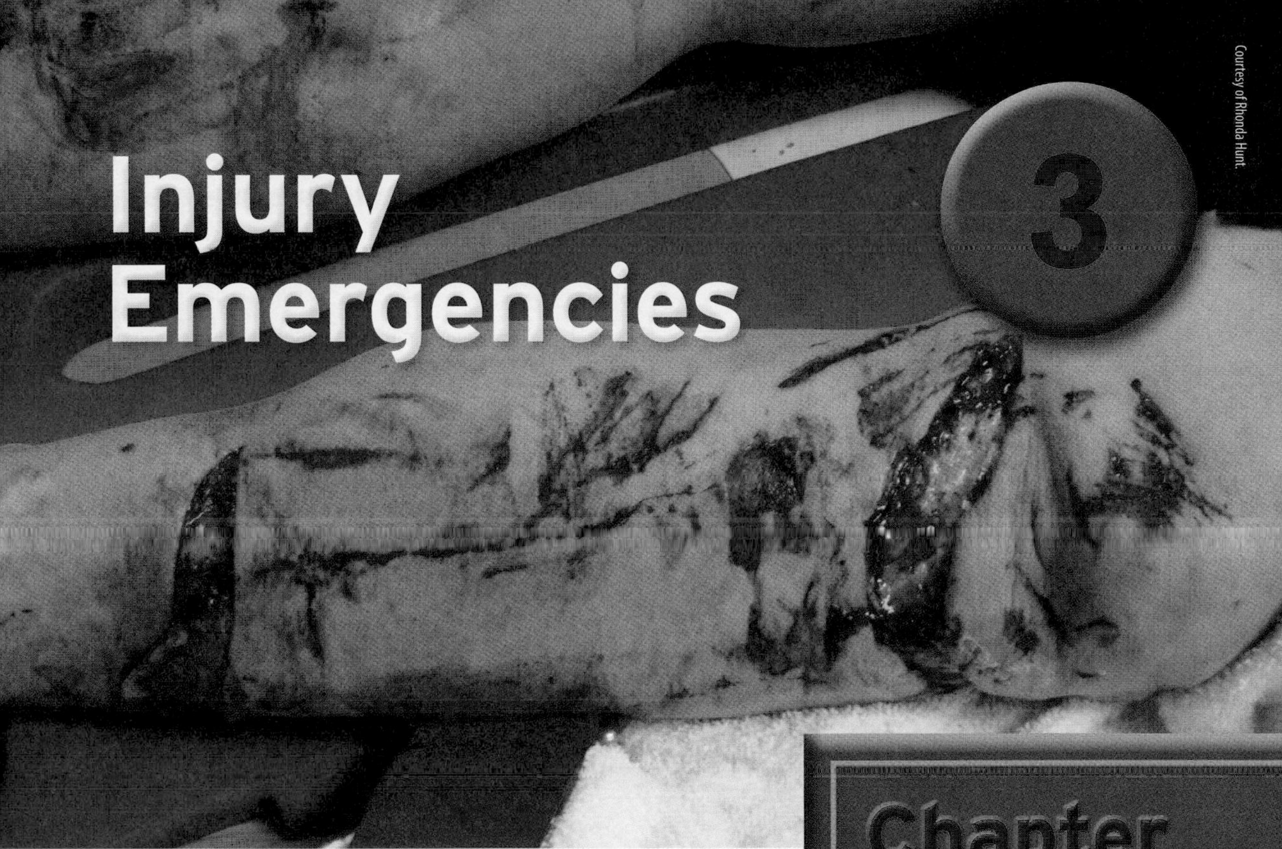

Injury Emergencies

3

Chapter at a glance

▶ Bleeding Control

Before helping, take the appropriate actions described on pages 5–6.

Avoid contact with blood by putting on disposable medical exam gloves. If gloves are unavailable, use a plastic bag, extra dressings, or clean cloths, or have the person apply pressure with his or her own hand, if possible.

Follow these steps to control bleeding Skill Sheet 3-1:

- Place a gauze dressing over the wound. If not available, use your gloved hand.
- Apply direct pressure using the flat part of the fingers or palm of the hand and/or a pressure bandage (eg, roller bandage) Figure 3-1.
- If the dressing becomes blood-soaked, add more dressings onto the first one and press harder and wider over the wound.
- **DO NOT** remove or apply any pressure on an impaled object.
- **DO NOT** apply pressure on a head wound (instead lightly press bulky dressings to the wound).

Skill Sheet

3-1 Bleeding Control

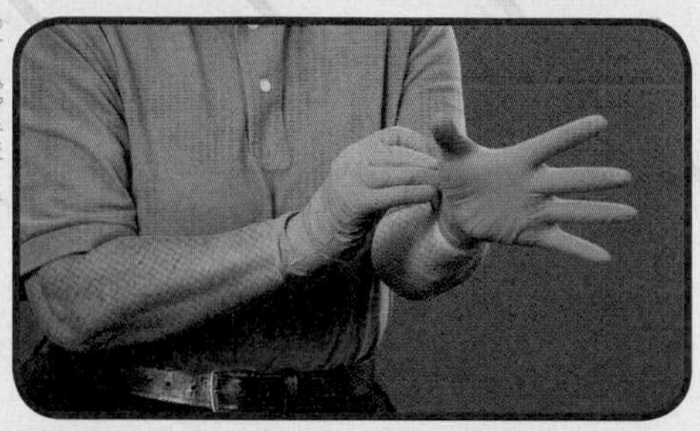

1. Put on gloves and expose the wound. If gloves are not available, improvise a barrier (eg, a plastic bag, plastic wrap, extra dressings or cloths). If those are not available, have the person apply pressure with his or her hand.

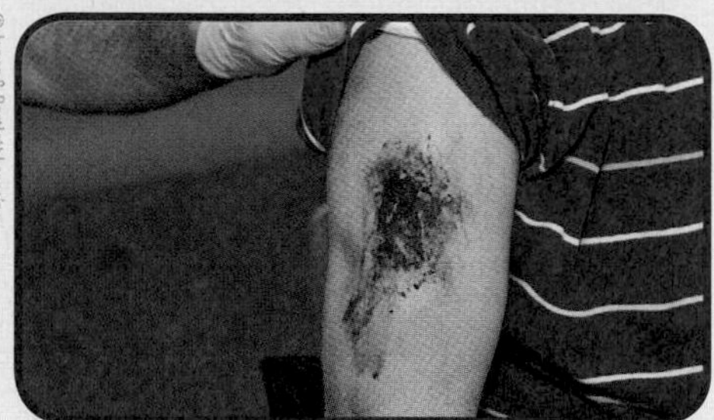

2. Cover the wound with a sterile or clean dressing.

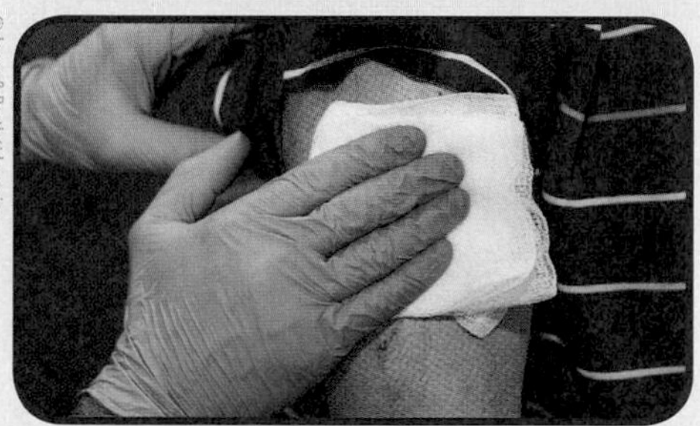

3. Apply direct pressure using the flat part of your fingers or palm of your hand to press on the wound until the bleeding stops. If you do not have a dressing, use your gloved hand.

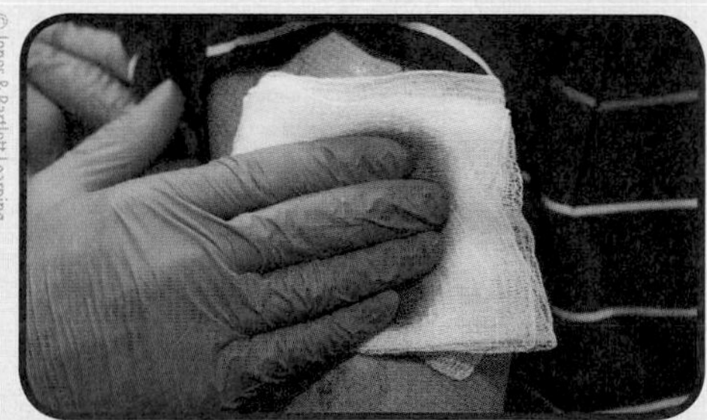

4. If the bleeding does not stop within 10 min, add more dressings onto the first one and press harder over a wider area. **DO NOT** remove blood-soaked dressings; instead add new dressings over the old ones.

Skill Sheet Continued

3-1 Bleeding Control

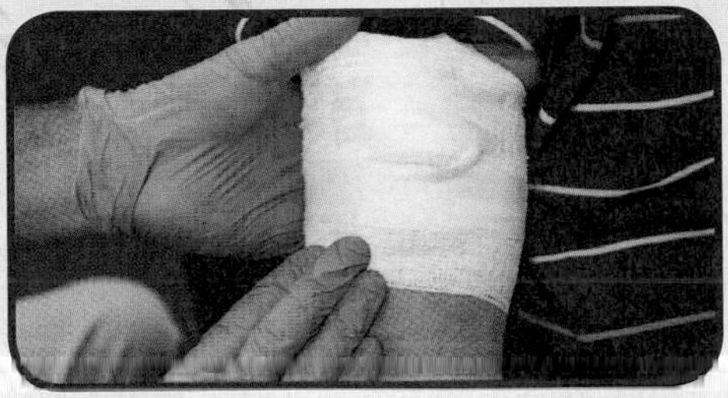

5. Apply a bandage firmly over the dressing to hold the dressing in place.

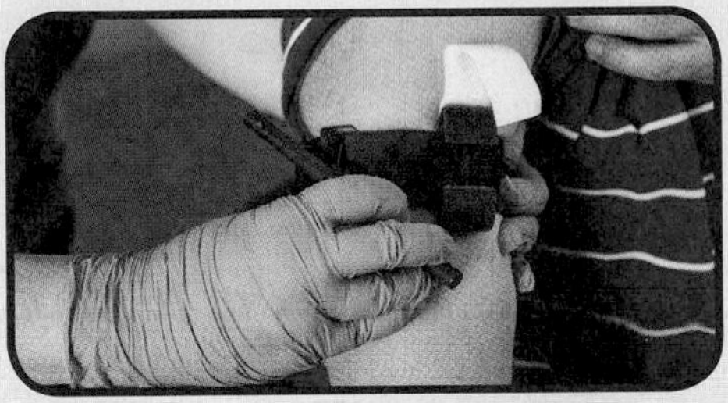

6. If the bleeding continues, call 9-1-1 if not already done. To save a life, consider using a tourniquet if severe bleeding (ie, spurting or flowing) from an arm or leg cannot be stopped by direct pressure (see Skill Sheet 3-2 and Skill Sheet 3-3).

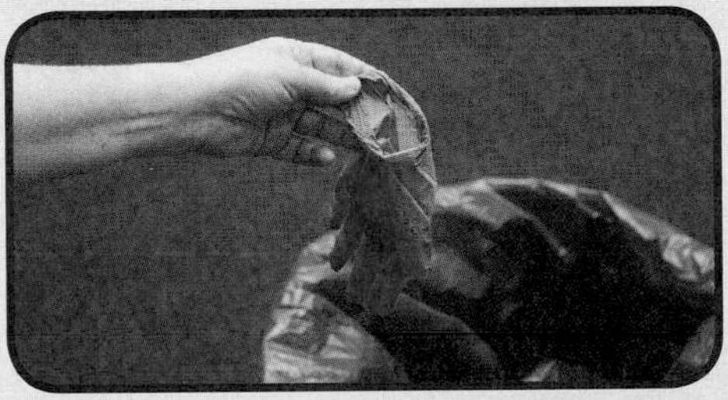

7. After the bleeding stops, properly dispose of the gloves and wash your hands.

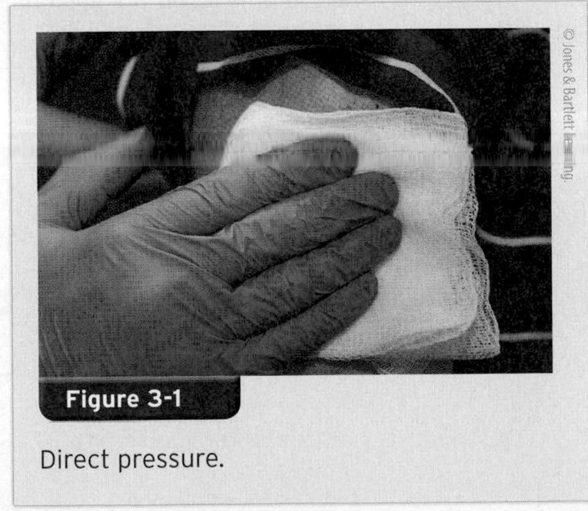

Figure 3-1

Direct pressure.

- **DO NOT** elevate an arm or leg or apply compression to a pressure point to control bleeding. There is no evidence these techniques are effective, and they may aggravate other injuries or delay the use of more effective methods. Applying compression on pressure points (ie, brachial, femoral arteries) can be difficult.

What to Look For	What to Do
Bleeding is controlled	1. Care for the wound. (Refer to pages 23-26.) 2. If needed, seek medical care for cleaning, stitches, or a tetanus immunization.
Bleeding continues	1. Apply a manufactured tourniquet 2 to 3 inches (5 to 7 cm) above the wound **Figure 3-2**. • Tourniquets are used only on arms and legs. • Tighten the tourniquet until the bleeding stops, then secure it in place. If bleeding continues, apply a second tourniquet near the first one. 2. Manufactured tourniquets appear to be better than those that are improvised **Skill Sheet 3-2**. If a manufactured tourniquet is not available, an improvised tourniquet can be applied **Skill Sheet 3-3**: • Wrap a band of soft material (eg, folded triangular bandage) twice around the arm or leg and about 2 to 3 inches (5 to 7 cm) above the wound. • **DO NOT** use narrow materials (eg, belt, rope, or string; tourniquet should be 2 to 4 inches [5 to 10 cm] wide), elastic materials, or bungee-type devices. • Tie a half or overhand knot on the arm or leg and place a short rigid object (eg, stick, screwdriver) over it. Then, tie a square knot over the rigid object. • Twist the rigid object until the bleeding stops. • Tie or tape the rigid object in place to keep the tourniquet from unwinding. 3. **DO NOT** cover, release, or remove a tourniquet. Write "TQ" (for tourniquet) and the time it was applied on a piece of tape, and stick it on the person's forehead.
Bleeding still continues	1. Apply a hemostatic dressing if: • Direct pressure is not effective in controlling bleeding. • A tourniquet is not available, is ineffective, or cannot be applied (eg, wound is on abdomen, chest, back). 2. Apply a hemostatic dressing in combination with direct pressure, followed by a pressure bandage. Certain hemostatic dressings have been proven to be effective and safe **Figure 3-3**. 3. Call 9-1-1 if it has not already been done.

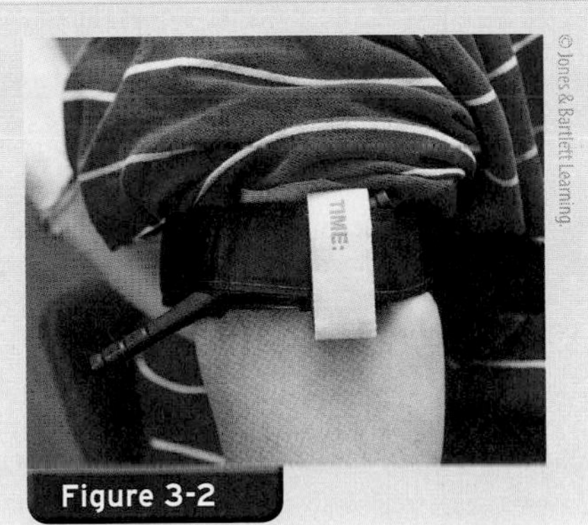

Figure 3-2

A tourniquet is a device wrapped tightly around an extremity to stop blood flow.

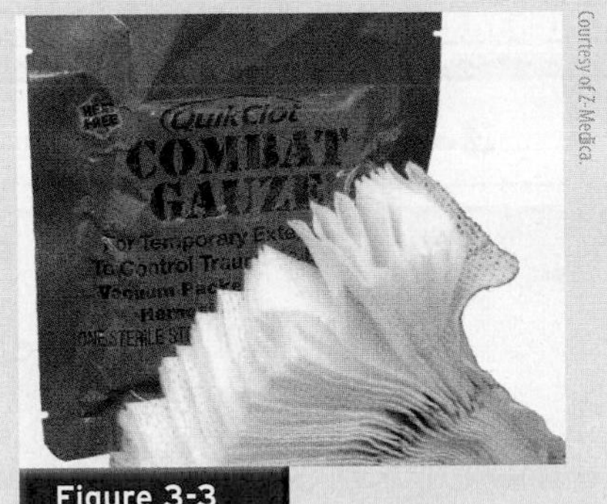

Figure 3-3

Hemostatic dressings are gauze-style dressings saturated with an agent that stops bleeding.

Skill Sheet

3-2 Applying a Manufactured Tourniquet

Apply a tourniquet to save a life when direct pressure cannot stop the bleeding (see Skill Sheet 3-1: Bleeding Control). Call 9-1-1 if it has not already been done.

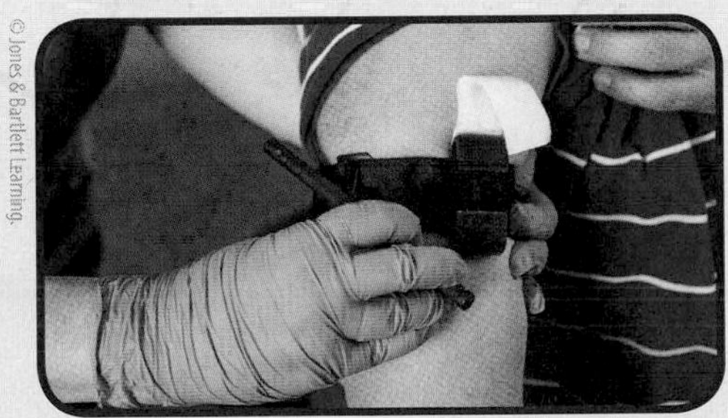

1. Apply the tourniquet firmly in place about 2 in. (5 cm) above the wound. **DO NOT** apply it anywhere other than an arm or leg. **DO NOT** apply it over a joint.

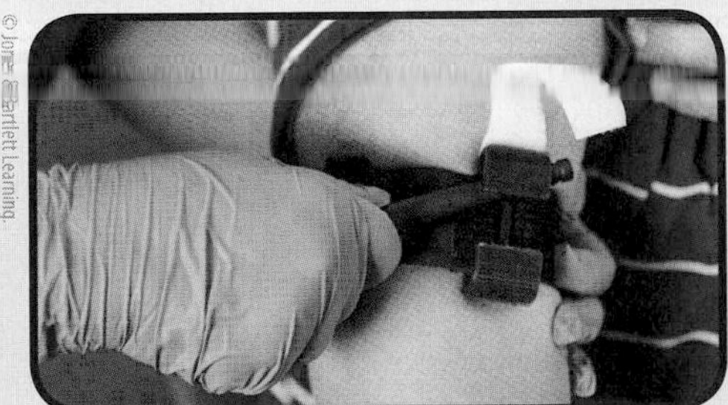

2. Tighten the tourniquet by twisting the rod until the bleeding stops. Secure the rod in place.

Skill Sheet Continued

3-2 Applying a Manufactured Tourniquet

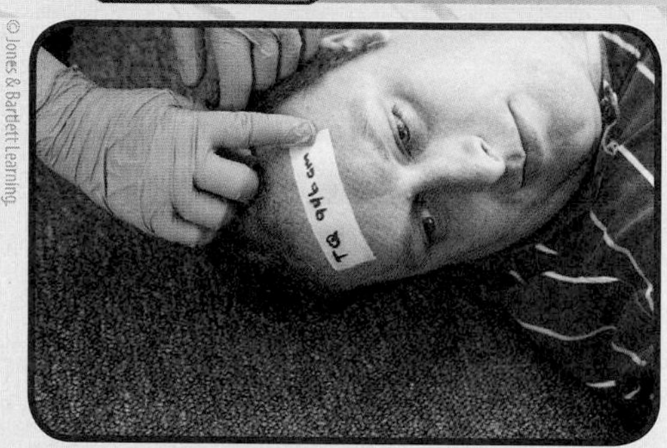

3. Write "TQ" (for tourniquet) and the time it was applied on a piece of tape, and stick it on the person's forehead. **DO NOT** cover a tourniquet. **DO NOT** release a tourniquet.

Skill Sheet

3-3 Applying an Improvised Tourniquet

Improvise a tourniquet to save a life when direct pressure cannot stop the bleeding (see Skill Sheet 3-1) and a manufactured tourniquet is not available. Call 9-1-1 if not already done.

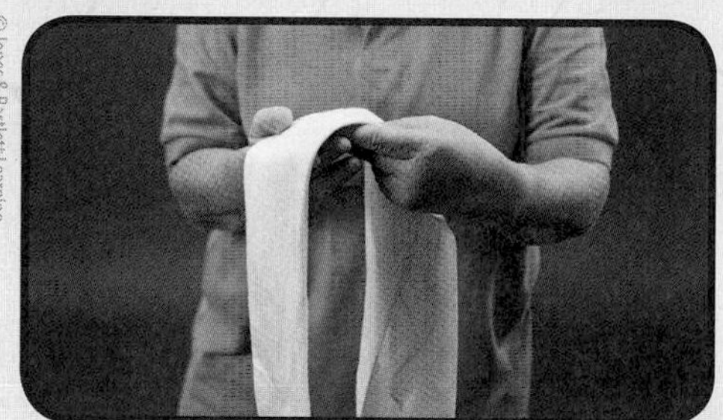

1. Use a folded triangle bandage, wide roller bandage, or similar cloth folded into a long band about 2 in. (5 cm) wide and several layers thick. **DO NOT** use narrow materials (eg, wire, rope, cord).

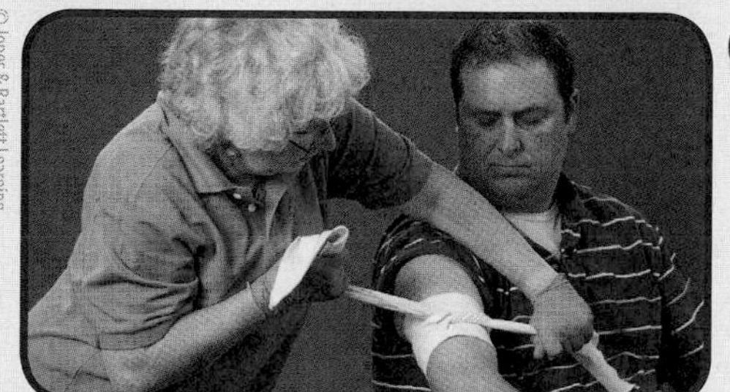

2. Wrap the band twice around the arm or leg about 2 in. (5 cm) above the wound and tie a knot (ie, overhand knot). Place padding underneath the band. **DO NOT** apply it anywhere other than the arm or leg. **DO NOT** apply it over a joint.

Skill Sheet Continued

3-3 Applying an Improvised Tourniquet

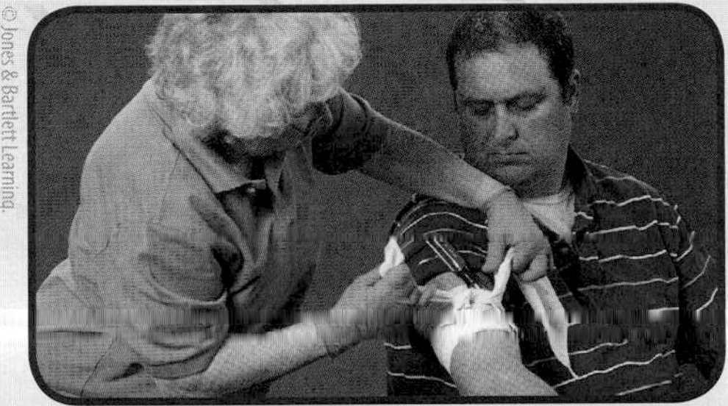

3. Place a short (6-8 in. [15-20 cm]) rigid object (eg, stick, screwdriver) onto the knot and then tie a square knot over the rigid object.

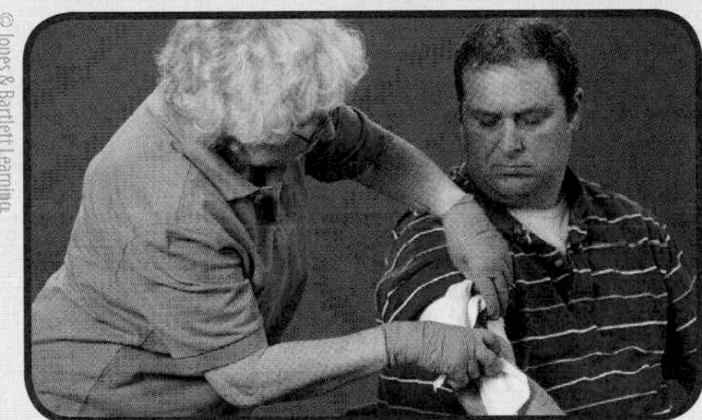

4. Twist the rigid object until the bleeding stops. Secure the rigid object in place with another cloth band or tape to prevent the tourniquet from untwisting.

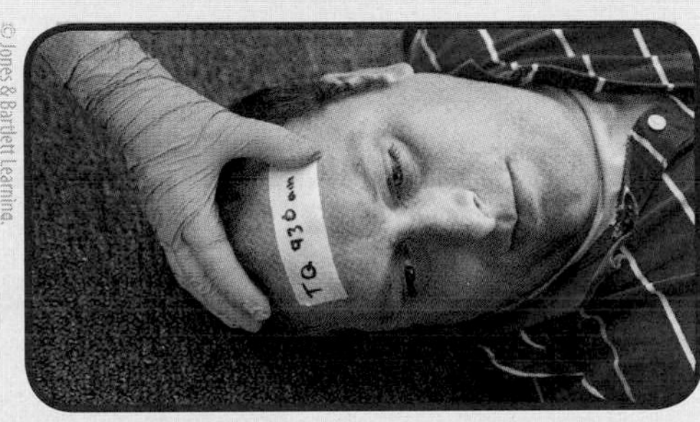

5. Write "TQ" (for tourniquet) and the time it was applied on a piece of tape and stick it on the person's forehead. **DO NOT** cover the tourniquet. **DO NOT** release a tourniquet.

▶ Wound Care

When possible, scrub your hands vigorously with soap and running water before and after cleaning a wound. If water is not available, use an alcohol hand sanitizer gel.

Shallow Wound

1. Gently wash inside and around the wound with warm or room-temperature running water and with or without soap. Cold water is as effective as warm water but is uncomfortable. If running water is not available, use any source of clean water.

Skill Sheet

3-4 Applying a Roller Bandage on a Forearm (Spiral Method)

Use a 2-in. (5-cm) roller bandage for an arm, or a 4-in. (10-cm) roller bandage for a leg.

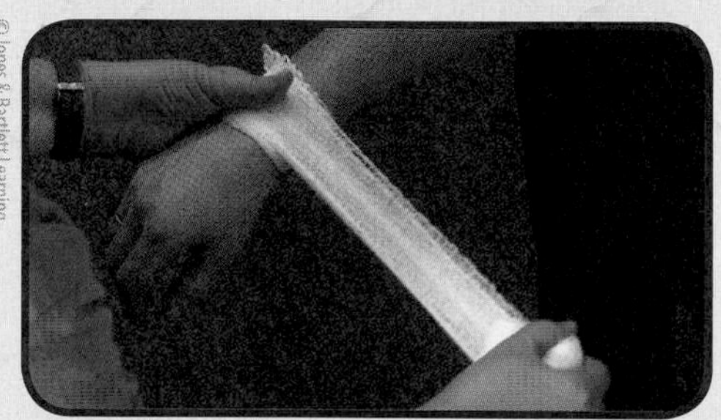

1. Start below and at the edge of the dressing. Make 2 straight anchoring turns with the bandage.

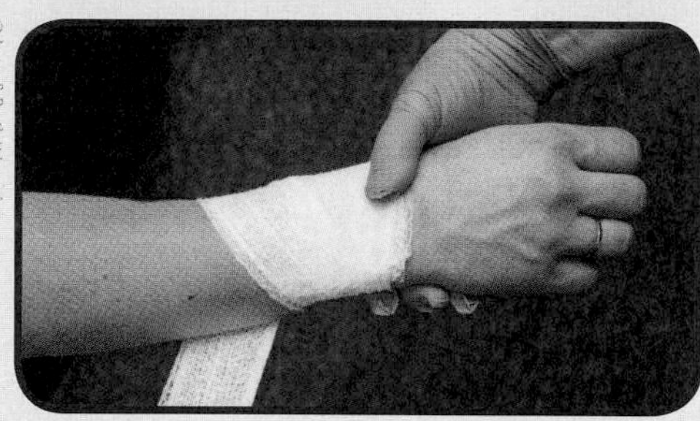

2. Wrap upward toward the wider part of the arm or leg to make the bandage more secure.

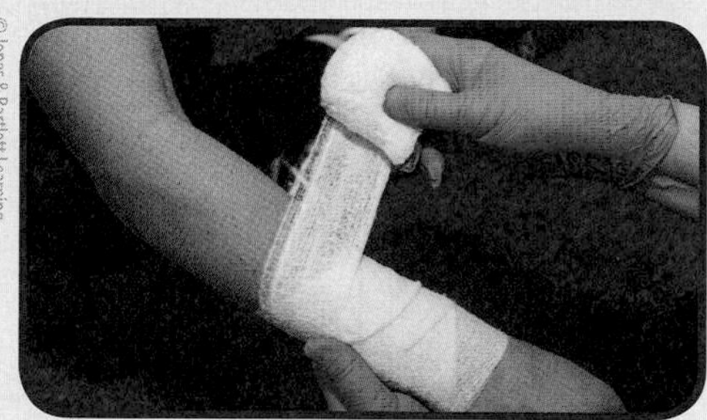

3. Make a series of criss-cross (figure-eight) turns, progressing up the arm or leg. Each turn should overlap the previous wrap.

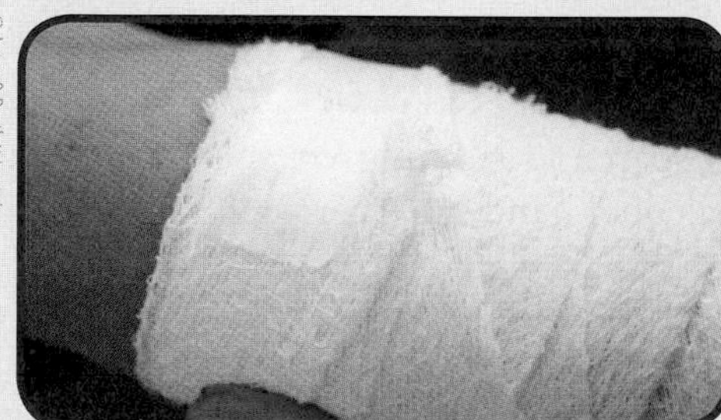

4. Finish with 2 straight turns and secure (ie, tape) the bandage.

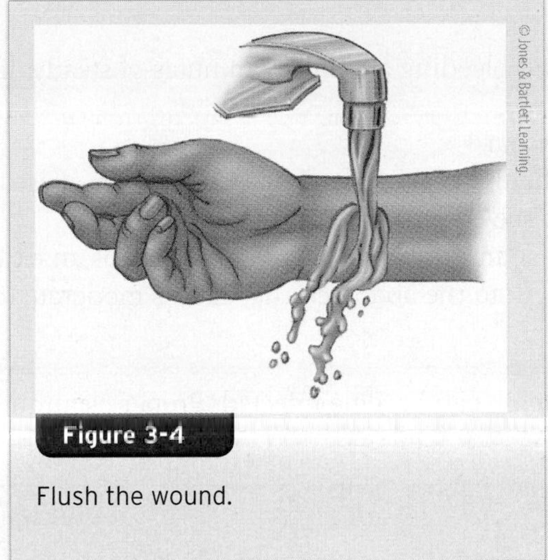

Figure 3-4

Flush the wound.

2. Flush with pressurized water (ie, from a faucet) inside the wound Figure 3-4. Pat the area dry.
3. If bleeding restarts, apply direct pressure.
4. Apply a thin layer of antibiotic ointment over the wound if the person is not sensitive to the medication. **DO NOT** apply hydrogen peroxide, alcohol, or iodine.
5. Cover the wound with a sterile or clean dressing and bandage.

Severe Wound

1. For a wound with a high risk of infection (eg, animal bite, very dirty or ragged wound, puncture wound), clean as best you can.
2. Cover with a sterile or clean dressing held in place by a bandage.
3. Care for shock; keep the person from getting chilled or overheated.

When to Seek Medical Care

The American College of Emergency Physicians says to seek medical care for any of the following:

- Long or deep cuts that need stitches
- Cuts over a joint
- Cuts from an animal or human bite
- Cuts that may impair function of a body area, such as an eyelid or lip
- Cuts that remove all the layers of the skin, such as slicing off the tip of a finger
- Cuts caused by metal objects or puncture wounds
- Cuts over a possible broken bone
- Cuts that are deep, jagged, or gaping open
- Cuts that have damaged underling nerves, tendons, or joints
- Cuts in which foreign materials, such as dirt, glass, metal, or chemicals, are embedded
- Cuts that show signs of infection, such as fever, swelling, redness, a pungent smell, pus, or fluid draining from the area
- Cuts that include problems with movement or sensation, or increased pain

Call 9-1-1 immediately if:

- The wound is still bleeding after a few minutes of steady, firm pressure with a cloth or bandage
- Signs of shock occur
- Breathing is difficult because of a cut to the neck or chest
- There is a cut to the eyeball
- There is a cut that amputates or partially amputates an extremity
- There is a deep cut to the abdomen that causes moderate to severe pain

Infected Wound

Any wound, large or small, can become infected. Proper cleaning can help prevent infections.

What to Look For	What to Do
• Swelling and redness around wound • Feeling of increased temperature compared to surrounding area (ie, wound feels warmer) • Throbbing pain • Pus discharge • Fever • Swelling of lymph nodes • One or more red streaks leading from the wound toward the heart (this is a serious sign that the infection is spreading)	1. Soak the wound in warm water, or apply warm, wet packs over the infected wound. Separate the wound edges to allow pus to escape. 2. Apply an antibiotic ointment. 3. Change the dressings several times a day. 4. Give pain medication. 5. Seek medical care if the infection becomes worse.

▶ Blisters

Before helping, take the appropriate actions described on pages 5–6.

The following procedures are for friction blisters Figure 3-5. **DO NOT** use these procedures for blisters related to poison ivy, burns, or frostbite.

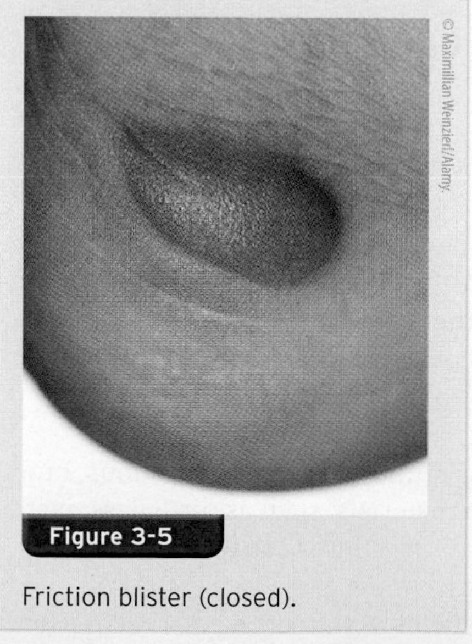

Figure 3-5

Friction blister (closed).

What to Look For	What to Do
Hot spot (painful, red area caused by rubbing)	1. Depending upon availability and the blister's location, relieve pressure on the area by applying one of the following: • Blister bandage (Blist-O-Ban) • Surgical tape (Micropore paper tape) • Elastic tape (Elastikon) 2. Trim and round the edges of the tape to prevent it from peeling off.
Blister that is closed and not very painful	Depending upon availability and the location of the blister, use the most appropriate method previously discussed.
Blister that is closed and very painful	1. Clean the blister and a needle with an alcohol pad. 2. Make several small holes at the base of the blister with the needle Figure 3-6. **DO NOT** make one large hole. Gently press the fluid out. **DO NOT** remove the blister roof unless it is torn. 3. Apply paper tape to protect the blister roof from being torn away when other overlying tape is removed. 4. Cover paper tape with elastic or adhesive tape. 5. Trim and round the edges of the tape to prevent it from peeling off. 6. Watch for signs of an infection.
Blister that is very painful and open or torn	1. Use scissors to carefully trim off the dead skin. 2. Place a blister pad (Spenco 2nd Skin) over the raw skin. 3. Cover the blister pad with paper tape. 4. Cover paper tape with elastic or adhesive tape. Trim and round the edges of the tape to prevent it from peeling off. 5. Watch for signs of an infection.

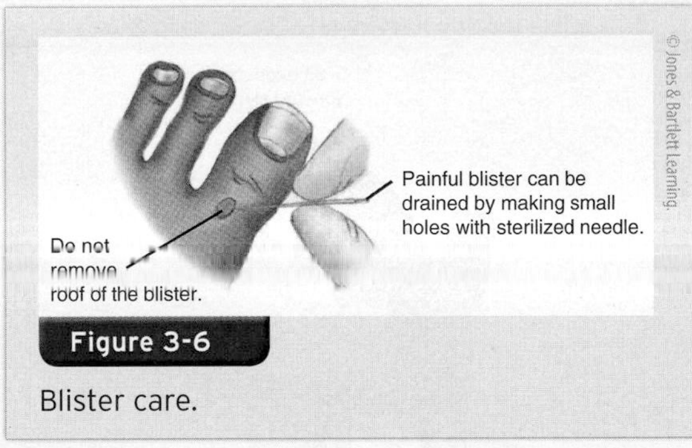

Figure 3-6

Blister care.

▶ Nose Injuries

Before helping, take the appropriate actions described on pages 5–6.

What to Look For	What to Do
Broken nose • Has been hit • May or may not be deformed	1. If bleeding, care for the nosebleed. 2. Apply an ice pack for 15 minutes. 3. Medical care can be delayed. 4. **DO NOT** try to straighten a crooked nose.
Nosebleed • Swelling • Bleeding • Difficulty breathing	1. If nose was hit, suspect a broken nose. 2. Have the person sit leaning slightly forward **Figure 3-7**. **DO NOT** tilt the head back or lie the person down. 3. Pinch the nostrils shut constantly for 10 minutes. Tell the person to breathe through the mouth and not swallow any blood. 4. If bleeding has not stopped, have the person gently blow his or her nose to get rid of ineffective blood clots. Pinch the nostrils together again for 10 minutes. 5. Try other methods in addition to nose pinching, such as applying an ice pack or spraying decongestant spray in nostrils. 6. Medical care is not usually needed. If bleeding reoccurs or if the nose is broken, seek medical care.
Foreign object in the nose (a medical condition mainly occurring to children)	Try one or more of the following methods to remove an object: 1. Have the person gently blow his or her nose while compressing the opposite nostril. 2. If an object is visible, pull it out with tweezers. **DO NOT** push the object deeper. 3. Have the person induce sneezing by sniffing pepper. 4. Seek medical care if the object cannot be removed.

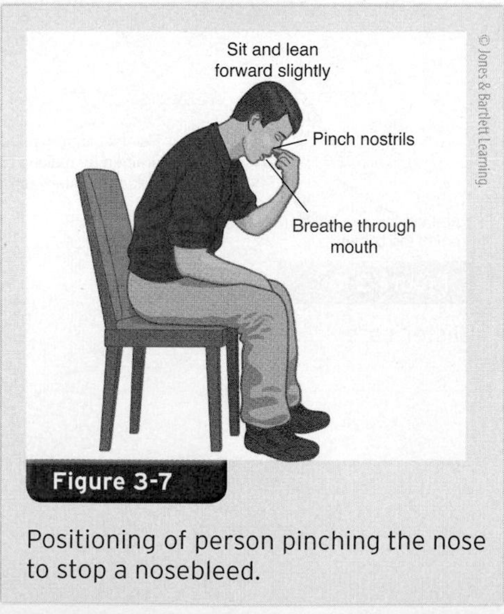

Figure 3-7

Positioning of person pinching the nose to stop a nosebleed.

▶ Tooth Injuries

Before helping, take the appropriate actions described on pages 5–6.

Seek dental care for all dental injuries—in most cases, as soon as possible.

What to Look For	What to Do
Toothache	1. Rinse the person's mouth with warm water. 2. Use dental floss to remove any trapped food. 3. Place an ice pack on the outside of the cheek to reduce swelling. 4. If available, use a cotton swab to paint the aching tooth with oil of cloves (eugenol). 5. **DO NOT** place aspirin on the aching tooth or gum tissue. 6. Give pain medication (eg, acetaminophen, ibuprofen). 7. Seek a dentist.
Broken tooth **Figure 3-8**	1. Collect all the tooth or teeth fragments. Depending upon the severity of injury, a dentist may be able to reattach them. 2. Rinse the person's mouth with warm water. 3. For swelling over the injured area, place an ice pack on the outside of the cheek. 4. For pain, have the person keep air exposure to a minimum by keeping the mouth closed. Additionally, consider providing pain medication, which should be swallowed. 5. If a jaw fracture is suspected, stabilize the jaw by wrapping a bandage under the chin and over the top of the head. 6. Seek a dentist as soon as possible. 7. Transport the fragments as you would a knocked-out tooth (see below).
Knocked-out (avulsed) tooth **Figure 3-9**	1. Attempt to reimplant tooth (only if it is a permanent [adult] tooth): • **DO NOT** touch the root. • If the tooth is dirty, rinse in bowl of warm water. **DO NOT** scrub or remove any of the attached tissue fragments. • Gently push the tooth down into the socket so the top is even with adjacent teeth. The person can bite down gently on gauze or a handkerchief placed between the teeth. 2. If unable to reimplant, keep the knocked-out tooth viable by storing it in a solution (listed in order of preference): • Hank's Balanced Salt Solution • Egg white • Coconut water • Whole milk If none of these are available, have the person spit saliva into a small container in which the tooth can be placed. **DO NOT** place the tooth in the mouth. **DO NOT** store it in water. 3. Seek a dentist as soon as possible.

(continued)

What to Look For	What to Do
Infected or abscessed tooth • Swelling of the gums around the affected tooth • Foul breath • Pain that is increased by tapping the tooth with something metal (eg, spoon handle)	1. Have the person rinse his or her mouth several times a day with warm water. 2. Give pain medication. **DO NOT** have the person suck an aspirin, and **DO NOT** place an aspirin on the tooth or gum tissue. 3. An ice pack on the cheek may help. 4. Use dental floss to remove any trapped food. 5. Seek a dentist.
Cavity—caused by decay or lost filling • Sensitivity to heat, cold, or sweets • Sensitivity to touch (Tap the tooth gently with something metal [eg, spoon handle] on the top and side. This increases the pain in the affected tooth.)	1. Have the person rinse his or her mouth with warm water. 2. Apply oil of cloves (eugenol) with a cotton swab to the cavity to deaden the pain. **DO NOT** apply any on the gums or lips, or inside the cheeks. 3. If available, apply a temporary filling with cavity dental filling paste. Other options include sugarless chewing gum, candle wax, or ski wax. 4. Seek a dentist.
Bleeding from mouth	1. Allow blood to drain out of the mouth. 2. For a bleeding tongue, put a dressing on the wound and apply pressure. 3. For a cut through a lip, place a rolled dressing between the lip and gum and press another dressing against the outer lip. 4. Seek medical care.

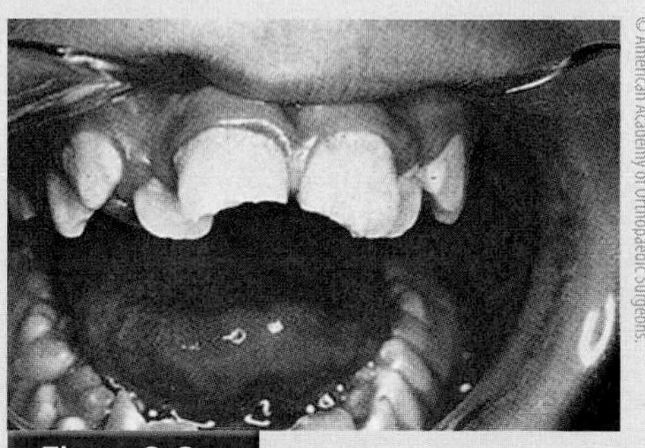

Figure 3-8

Broken teeth.

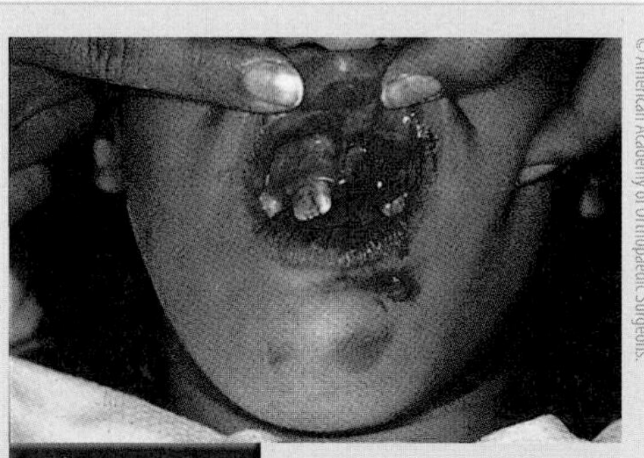

Figure 3-9

Knocked-out tooth.

▶ Eye Injuries

Before helping, take the appropriate actions described on pages 5–6.

Seek medical care for all eye injuries. **DO NOT** assume that an eye injury is minor. Some eye injuries require calling 9-1-1 as soon as possible. Medical care should also be sought for double vision, pain, or reduced vision.

What to Look For	What to Do
Blow to eye	1. Apply an ice pack around the eye for 15 minutes. **DO NOT** place the pack on the eye. 2. Have the person keep the eyes closed. 3. Seek medical care.
Loose object in eye	Try, in order, each of the following steps: 1. Have the person blink the eye several times. 2. Pull upper eyelid out and over lower lid. 3. Gently irrigate the eye with clean, warm water. 4. Lift eyelid up and over a cotton swab. If object is seen, remove it with the corner of a wet gauze pad. 5. If successful, medical care is usually not needed unless there is continued pain or itching to the eye.
Object stuck in eye	1. **DO NOT** remove the object. 2. For a long object, place padding around the object to stabilize against movement, and place a paper cup or similar object over the object for protection. 3. For a short object, place a doughnut-shaped pad around the eye, and wrap a bandage around the head to hold the pad in place. 4. Cover both eyes; movement of the uninjured eye will cause movement of the injured eye. 5. Keep the person flat on his or her back. 6. Call 9-1-1 as soon as possible.
Cut on the eyeball	1. **DO NOT** apply pressure to the eye. 2. Cover both eyes with gauze pads, and lightly wrap a bandage around the head to hold the pads in place. 3. Call 9-1-1 or drive to a medical facility as soon as possible.
Chemical, smoke, or other irritant in eye	1. Hold the eye wide open; flush with warm water for at least 15 minutes or until emergency medical services (EMS) arrives. If tap water is not available, normal saline or other eye irrigation solution may be used Figure 3-10. 2. The eye(s) may need to be loosely bandaged. 3. For a chemical eye injury, contact the poison control center (1-800-222-1222). If not available, seek medical care as soon as possible or call 9-1-1.

(continued)

What to Look For	What to Do
Burns caused by light (from looking at sunlight or reflection off of snow or water); these burns may not be painful at first but become very painful hours later.	1. Cover both eyes with moist, cool cloths. 2. Give pain medication if needed. 3. Seek medical advice.

▶ Ear Injuries

Before helping, take the appropriate actions described on pages 5–6.

What to Look For	What to Do
Objects stuck in an ear	1. **DO NOT** use tweezers or try to pry an object out. 2. Seek medical care to remove the object. Except for disc batteries and live insects, few foreign bodies must be removed immediately. 3. For a live insect in the ear canal, shine a small light into the ear. The insect may crawl out toward the light; if it does not, pour warm water into the ear and then drain it. This may drown the insect; regardless of whether it is dead or alive, it should wash out. When draining the water, turn the head to the side. If the insect cannot be removed, seek medical care.
Fluids coming from the ear (blood or clear fluid draining from the ear may indicate a skull fracture)	1. **DO NOT** attempt to stop flow of blood or clear fluid (known as cerebrospinal fluid [CSF]), with or without blood, coming from an ear. Doing so could increase pressure on the brain, causing permanent damage. 2. Place a sterile gauze dressing over the ear and loosely bandage it in place to prevent bacteria getting into the brain. 3. Stabilize the head and neck against movement. 4. Call 9-1-1.

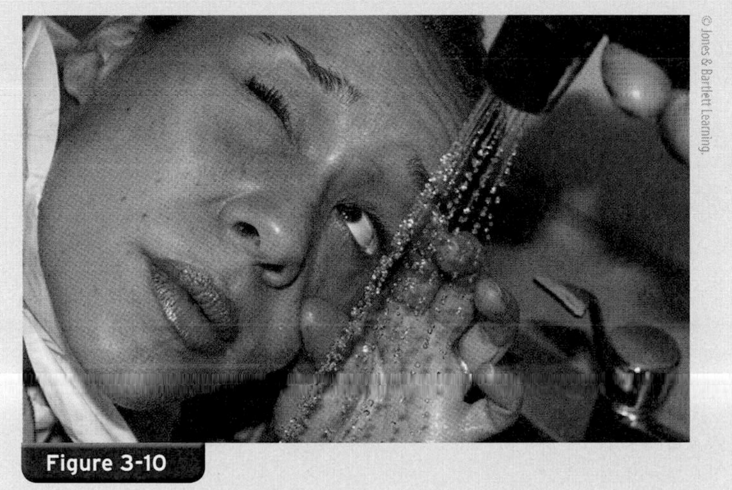

Figure 3-10

For chemical burns, rinse the eyes with water, with the injured eye on the bottom to avoid exposing the uninjured eye to the chemical.

▶ Impaled (Embedded) Object

Before helping, take the appropriate actions described on pages 5–6.

What to Look For	What to Do
Sliver (also referred to as a splinter)	1. Remove with tweezers (may need to use a sterile needle to tease the sliver into a better position for removal). 2. Wash the area with soap and water. 3. Apply antibiotic ointment. 4. Apply an adhesive bandage.
Large object (such as a knife, pencil, steel rod) Figure 3-11	1. **DO NOT** remove or move the object. 2. Stabilize the object with bulky dressings or padding placed around the base of the object to keep it from moving. 3. If bleeding, apply direct pressure around the base of the object. **DO NOT** apply pressure on the object or on the skin next to the sharp edges of the object. 4. If necessary, reduce the length or weight of the object by cutting or breaking it. 5. Call 9-1-1 if it has not already been done.

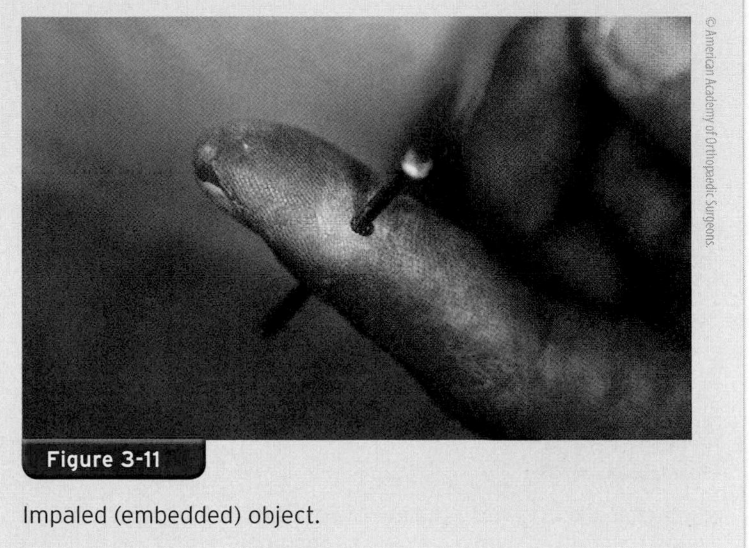

Figure 3-11

Impaled (embedded) object.

Amputations and Avulsions

Before helping, take the appropriate actions described on pages 5–6.

Control the bleeding by applying direct pressure and firmly securing a pressure bandage over the stump or area of avulsion. If the bleeding continues, apply a tourniquet or a hemostatic dressing. Treat for shock by lying the person flat and covering him or her.

What to Look For	What to Do
Amputation Figure 3-12	1. Call 9-1-1. 2. If a body part is amputated, immediate action is needed for reattachment. Amputated body parts that are left uncooled for more than 6 hours have little chance of survival. 3. Control bleeding by using pressure; if unsuccessful, apply a tourniquet or a hemostatic dressing, if available. 4. Care for the amputated part: • Wrap the severed part in a sterile gauze or a clean cloth that has been wet with water (make sure the excess water has been squeezed out). • Put the wrapped part in a waterproof container (eg, plastic bag, plastic wrap). • Keep the part cool by placing the wrapped part in a container of ice. **DO NOT** bury the part in the ice or allow it to touch the ice. **DO NOT** submerge it in water. • Send the part to the medical facility with the injured person. 5. If the amputated part was not found, ask others to search for it and, if located, to take it to the medical facility where the person is going.

What to Look For	What to Do
Avulsion (a flap of skin torn loose but still attached and hanging from the body) Figure 3-13	1. Gently move the skin back to its normal position. 2. Cover with a sterile or clean dressing and apply pressure. 3. If bleeding continues, apply a tourniquet or a hemostatic dressing, if available.

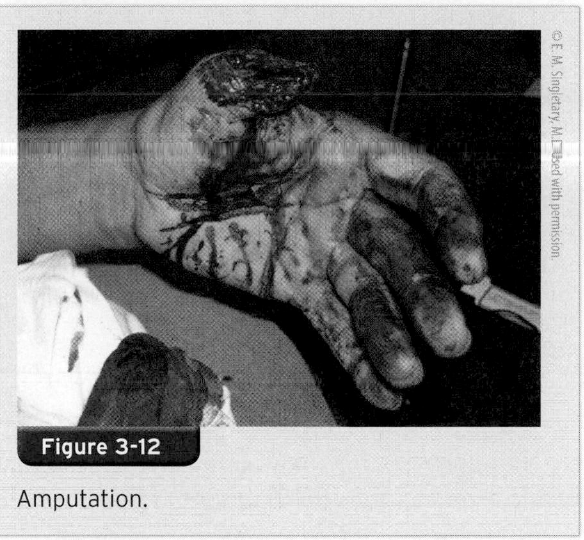

Figure 3-12

Amputation.

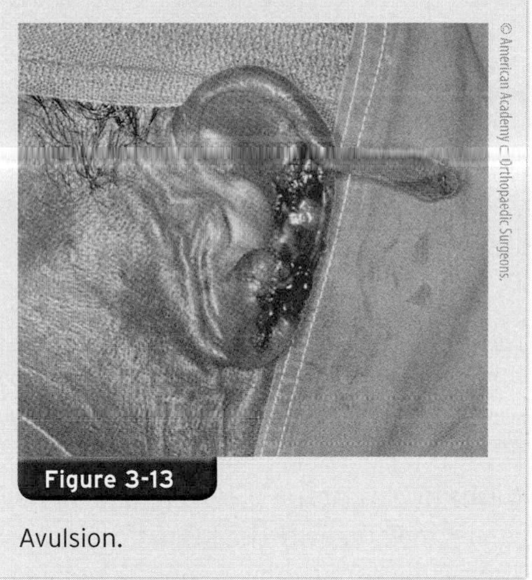

Figure 3-13

Avulsion.

▶ Head Injuries

Before helping, take the appropriate actions described on pages 5–6.

Suspect a spinal cord injury in a person with a head injury (see pages 37–39).

What to Look For	What to Do
Scalp wound	1. Control bleeding by pressing on wound. Replace any skin flap to its original position and apply pressure. Another option is applying an ice pack or instant cold pack to control bleeding. 2. If you suspect a skull fracture, **DO NOT** apply excessive pressure; this may push bone pieces into the brain. Press on the edges of the wound to help control bleeding. 3. Apply a dry, sterile or clean dressing. 4. Keep the head and shoulders raised if no spinal injury is suspected. 5. If bleeding continues, **DO NOT** remove the first blood-soaked dressing; instead, add another dressing over it. 6. Call 9-1-1 if: • The wound is extensive. • There is significant facial damage. • Signs of concussion occur (eg, nausea and vomiting, headache, drowsiness).

Skull Fracture

What to Look For	What to Do
• Pain • Skull deformity • Bleeding from an ear or the nose • Leakage of clear, watery fluid from an ear or the nose (CSF) • Discoloration around the eyes or behind the ears that appears several hours after the injury • Unequal-sized pupils of the eye • Heavy scalp bleeding (skull and/or brain tissue may be exposed) • Penetrating or impaled object	1. Apply a sterile or clean dressing over the wound and hold it in place with gentle pressure. Harder pressure can be applied on the edges of the wound to avoid pressing bone pieces into the brain. 2. Control bleeding by pressing on the edges of the wound and gently on the center of it. A doughnut-shaped pad is useful in applying pressure around the edges of a suspected skull fracture Figure 3-14. 3. Call 9-1-1. 4. *Cautions:* • **DO NOT** move the head, neck, or spine. • **DO NOT** clean the wound. • **DO NOT** remove an embedded object. • **DO NOT** stop blood or clear fluid that is draining from an ear or the nose. • **DO NOT** press on the fractured area.

Brain Injury (Concussion)

A concussion is a type of traumatic brain injury caused by a bump, blow, or jolt to the head that can change the way the brain normally works. Most concussions (80% to 90%) resolve within 7 to 10 days, but some people take much longer to recover.

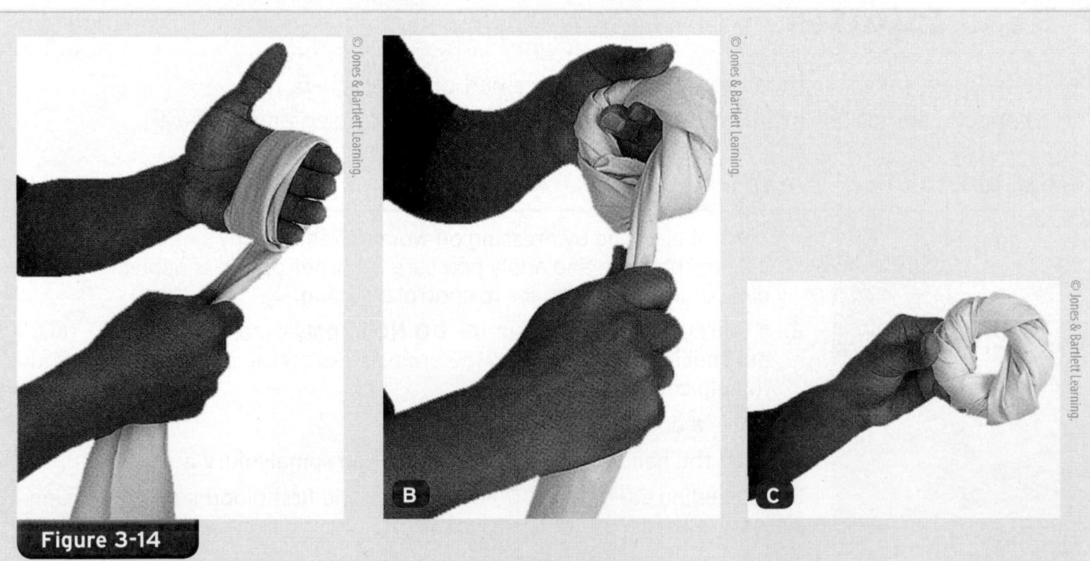

Figure 3-14

Make a "doughnut" for skull fracture-related bleeding and for eye protection when a short object is embedded. **A.** Using a triangular bandage or clean cloth, wrap about half the length into a circle large enough to surround the injured area. **B.** Pass the tail thorough the hole repeatedly to form a spiral. **C.** The completed dressing should have a hole large enough to prevent pressure on the injured area.

What to Look For

Recognition of a concussion is difficult. The following signs or symptoms may worsen over minutes or hours:

- Behavior or personality changes
- Blank stare/dazed look
- Changes to balance, coordination, and reaction time
- Delayed or slowed spoken or physical responses
- Disorientation, memory loss (confused about date/location)
- Loss of responsiveness (occurs in fewer than 10% of concussions)
- Slurred/unclear speech
- Difficulty controlling emotions
- Vomiting
- Headache
- Fuzzy or blurry vision
- Nausea
- Dizziness
- Sensitivity to noise or light

What to Do

1. If unresponsive, check for breathing. If breathing stops, call 9-1-1 and give cardiopulmonary resuscitation (CPR). (See pages 99-103.)
2. If a neck injury is suspected, or if the person is unresponsive:
   - **DO NOT** move the head, neck, or spine.
   - Call 9-1-1.
3. Seek medical care as soon as possible if the person:
   - Looks very drowsy or cannot be awakened
   - Has one pupil (the black part in the middle of the eye) that is larger than the other
   - Has a seizure
   - Cannot recognize people or places
   - Becomes more and more confused, restless, or agitated
   - Exhibits unusual behavior
   - Becomes unresponsive
   - Has a headache that gets worse and/or does not go away
   - Has repeated vomiting or nausea
   - Has slurred speech
4. Following the injury, the person should:
   - Get plenty of sleep at night and rest during the day.
   - Avoid visual and sensory stimuli, including video games and loud music.
   - Ease into normal activities slowly, not all at once.
   - Avoid strenuous physical activities that increase the heart rate or require a lot of concentration.
   - Avoid driving, cycling, operating machinery, or playing sports until assessed by a health care provider.
   - Avoid anything that could cause another blow to the head or body.
   - **DO NOT** use aspirin or anti-inflammatory medications such as ibuprofen or naproxen because of the risk of bleeding. (Acetaminophen can be used for postconcussion headaches.)

▶ Spinal Injury

Before helping, take the appropriate actions described on pages 5–6.

Suspect a spinal injury (includes neck, back, hip, or pelvis), if a person:

- Was in a motor vehicle crash involving ejection, a rollover, high speeds, or pedestrians
- Was involved in other types of motorized vehicle crashes (eg, motorcycle, scooter, all-terrain vehicle, snowmobile)

- Was involved in a bicycle or skateboard crash
- Fell greater than his or her standing height, especially if older
- Dove into shallow water
- Received a hit or blow to the head

Fully stabilizing a responsive person may not always be necessary; doing so can be difficult, impractical, impossible, or dangerous to the person. Injured people can be classified as either reliable or unreliable. A *reliable* person meets the following criteria:

- Alert, knows name and where he or she is
- Not intoxicated by drugs/alcohol
- Calm, cooperative
- Lack of an additional painful injury that could distract from the pain of a spinal injury

An *unreliable* person meets one or more of the following criteria:

- Unresponsive or altered mental status
- Intoxicated by drugs/alcohol
- Combative, confused
- Has an additional painful injury that could distract from the pain of a spinal injury

What to Look For	What to Do

A reliable person with signs of spinal injury:
• Reports of back pain and leg numbness and tingling
• Tenderness/pain when you run fingers all the way down spine (if possible). (Press each bump of vertebrae and press on depressions produced on each side when you touch or push on the spine bones.)
• Failure of the following tests for sensation and movement (test all four extremities):
  • Upper body:
    - Pinch several fingers while the person has his or her eyes closed, and ask, "Can you feel this?" and "Which finger am I touching?"
    - Ask, "Can you wiggle your fingers?"
    - Have the person squeeze your hand.
  • Lower body:
    - Pinch toes while the person has his or her eyes closed, and ask, "Can you feel this?" and "Which toe am I touching?"
    - Ask, "Can you wiggle your toes?"
    - Have the person push and pull a foot against your hand.
	1. Call 9-1-1. Wait for trained rescuers with proper equipment.
	2. **DO NOT** attempt to move the person. Leave the person in the position in which found. Tell the person to remain as still as possible. Consider moving a person only for the following: to provide CPR, to open a blocked airway, to control life-threatening bleeding, or to reach a safe location.
	3. Apply spinal stabilization by placing your hands on both sides of the head with the palms over the ears **Figure 3-15**.
	4. **DO NOT** apply a cervical (neck) collar **Figure 3-16**.
	5. Cover to prevent heat loss.

What to Look For	What to Do
A reliable person without signs of a spinal injury: • Alert, not intoxicated, and no distracting injuries • No report of neck pain or neurologic symptoms (eg, tingling, numbness) • No neck tenderness when felt, no loss of sensation when fingers and toes are pinched, and able to move the fingers and toes	1. An injured person without signs of a spinal injury does not require spinal stabilization. 2. Treat other injuries (eg, wounds, bruises, fractures).
An unreliable person with signs of a spinal injury (see examples previously discussed)	1. Assume a spinal injury exists. 2. Use the methods previously discussed to stabilize the person.

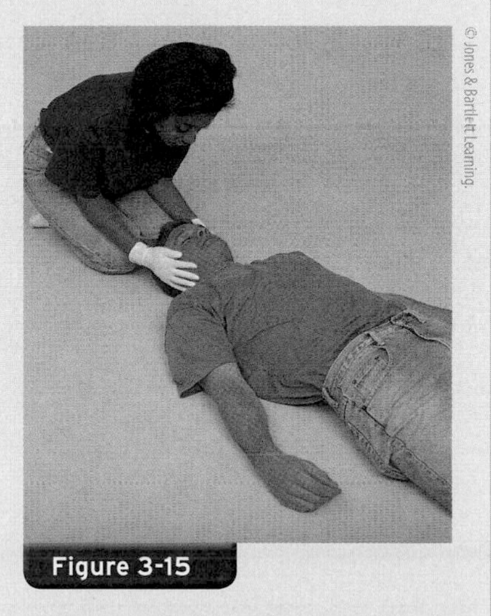

Figure 3-15

You can maintain spinal stabilization by using your hands.

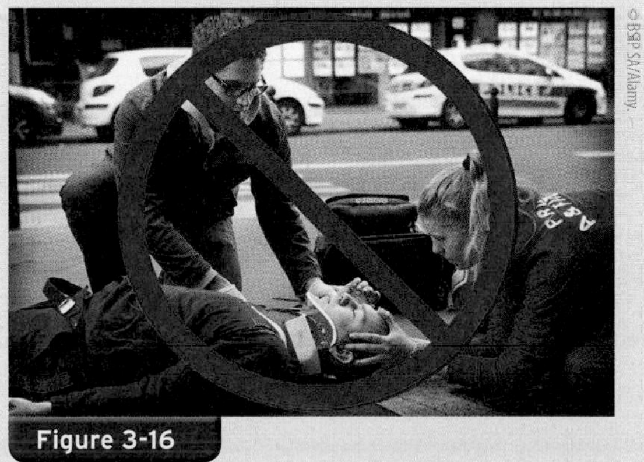

Figure 3-16

DO NOT place a cervical neck collar on a person with a suspected spinal injury.

▶ Chest Injuries

Before helping, take the appropriate actions described on pages 5–6.

Chest injuries can involve broken bones, penetrating injuries, and open or closed wounds. For all chest injuries, look for the following:

- DOTS: Deformity, Open wounds, Tenderness, and Swelling
- Abnormal breathing rate and/or sounds (eg, gurgling)
- Guarding (protecting an area during moving or touching)

Rib Fractures

What to Look For	What to Do
• Sharp pain when the person takes deep breaths, coughs, or moves • Guarding • Tenderness • Shallow breathing as a result of pain that occurs from normal or deep breathing • Bruising of skin over the injury (usually occurs along the side of the chest)	1. Help the person find a comfortable position. 2. Stabilize the chest by: • Having the person hold a pillow or other similarly soft material against the area, or • Placing arm on the injured side in a sling and binder (swathe) if necessary for pain control. 3. **DO NOT** apply tight bandages around the chest. 4. Give pain medication. 5. Have the person cough and take deep breaths, even if it hurts, a few times every hour to prevent pneumonia. 6. Call 9-1-1.

Flail Chest

A flail chest happens when several ribs in the same area are broken in more than one place.

What to Look For	What to Do
• Area over the injury moving in a direction opposite to that of the rest of the chest wall during breathing • Very painful and difficult breathing • Bruising of skin over the injury • Same signs as for rib fractures	1. Stabilize the chest by: • Placing a pillow or similarly soft material against area or arm on the injured side in a sling and binder (swathe), and • Placing the person on his or her injured side with a blanket or similarly soft material underneath the person. 2. **DO NOT** apply tight bandages around the chest. 3. Call 9-1-1.

Penetrating Object in Chest

What to Look For	What to Do
Impaled object (usually easy to see)	1. Stabilize the object in place with bulky dressings or clothes. **DO NOT** try to remove the object. 2. Call 9-1-1.

Open Chest Wound

What to Look For	What to Do
• Blood bubbling out of a chest wound during exhalation • Sucking sound heard during inhalations	1. Leave the wound exposed to air without a dressing or any airtight material. 2. **DO NOT** cover an open chest wound unless using direct pressure and a dry gauze dressing to control bleeding. If the dressing becomes blood-soaked, replace it to avoid trapping air in the chest, which may result in death. 3. Call 9-1-1.

▶ Abdominal Injuries

Before helping, take the appropriate actions described on pages 5–6.

DO NOT give anything to eat or drink. Position the person on his or her back with the knees bent if it does not cause pain. Treat for shock and keep the person from getting chilled or overheated.

What to Look For	What to Do
Penetrating object	1. **DO NOT** remove a penetrating object. 2. Stabilize the object against movement. 3. Call 9-1-1.
Protruding organs	1. **DO NOT** try to push protruding organs back into the abdomen. 2. **DO NOT** touch organs. 3. Cover them with a moist, clean dressing **Figure 3-17**. 4. Call 9-1-1.
Hard blow to abdomen	1. Roll the person onto one side and expect vomiting. 2. Monitor for signs of possible internal injuries, including: • Pain that gradually increases and may become severe. • Pain that markedly increases with slight movements. • Abdomen is very tender to touch. • Blood in vomit or bowel movement. • Bruising of the abdominal skin. 3. Call 9-1-1.

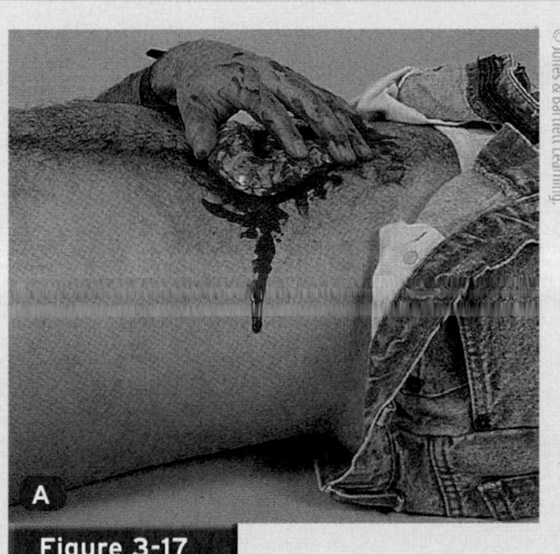

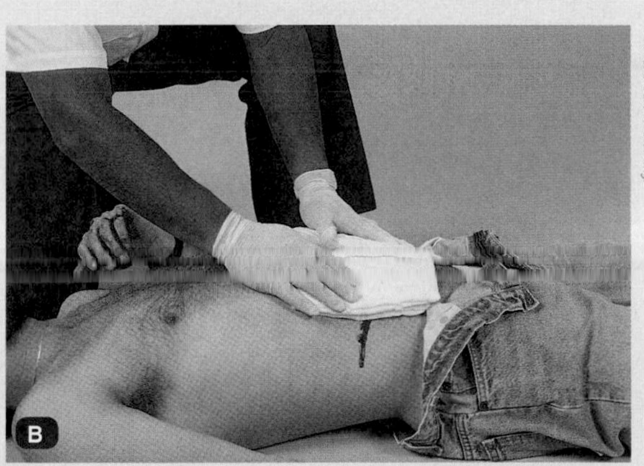

Figure 3-17

A. Protruding organs. **B.** Cover protruding organs with a moist, clean dressing.

▶ Bone, Joint, and Muscle Injuries

Before helping, take the appropriate actions described on pages 5–6.

For all bone, joint, and muscle injuries, use the RICE procedure Skill Sheet 3-5:

R = *Rest.* **DO NOT** use the injured part.
I = *Ice.* Apply an ice pack for 20 minutes (or 10 minutes if uncomfortable) every 2 to 3 hours during the first 24 to 48 hours following the injury.
C = *Compression.* Apply an elastic bandage when not applying ice.
E = *Elevation.* Keep the injured part raised higher than the heart as much as possible.

Skill Sheet

3-5 RICE Procedure for Bone, Joint, and Muscle Injuries

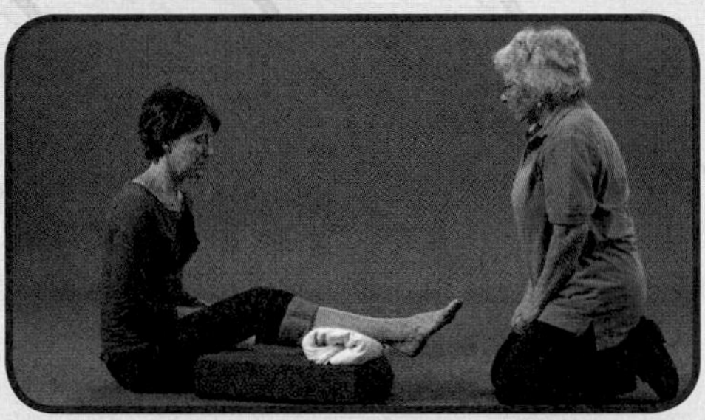

1 **R = Rest**
DO NOT use or move the body part.

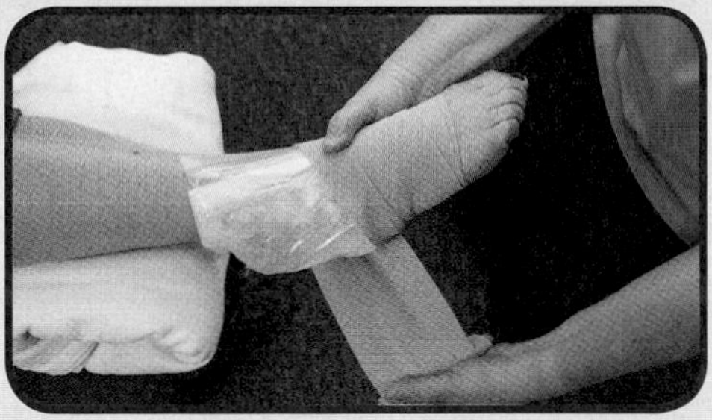

2 **I = Ice**
Apply cold for 20 min (or 10 min if uncomfortable) every 2-3 h during the first 24-48 h. Put crushed or cubed ice in a plastic bag and place a paper towel or thin cloth between the ice pack and skin for protection or put ice wrapped in a damp towel.

Skill Sheet Continued

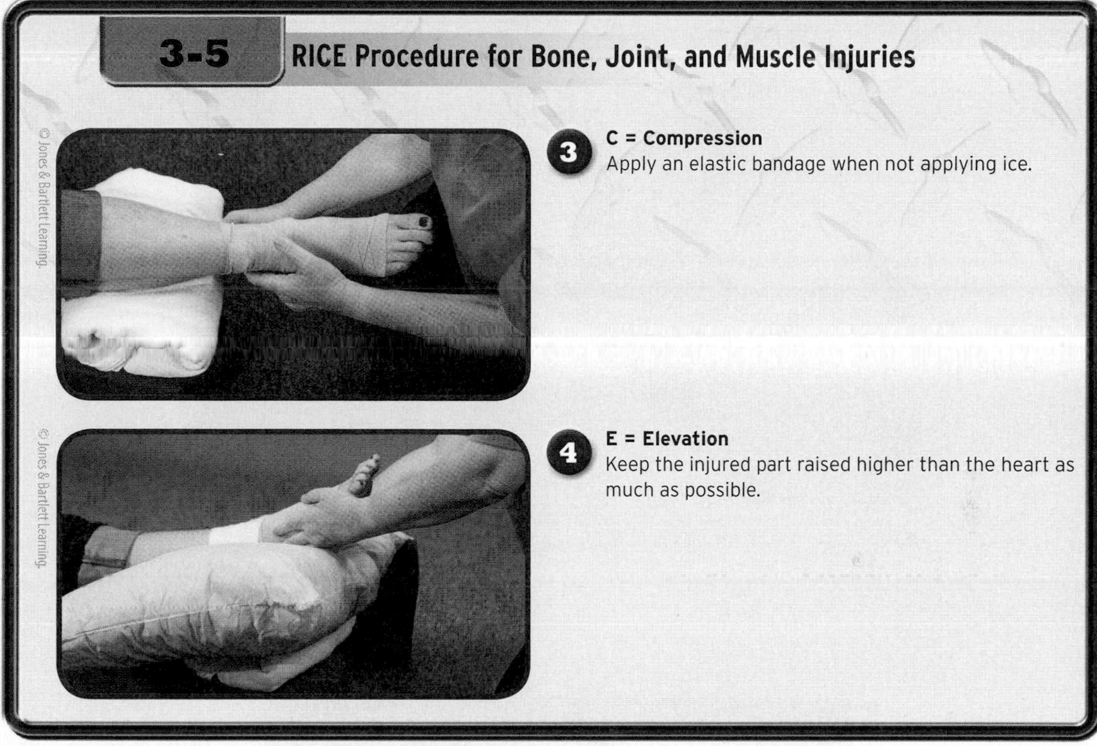

Bone Injuries (Fractures)

It may be difficult to tell whether a bone is broken. When in doubt, treat the injury as a broken bone. All broken bones need medical care, even if calling 9-1-1 is not necessary.

What to Look For

DOTS:

- **D**eformity (Compare the injured part with the uninjured part on the other side **Figure 3-18**)
- **O**pen wound **Figure 3-19**
- **T**enderness and pain (A useful technique for detecting a fracture is to gently feel, touch, or press along the length of the bone; a person's report of tenderness or pain can indicate a fracture.)
- **S**welling that happens rapidly

What to Do

1. Hold the part when transporting a short distance to a medical facility or until EMS arrives. If EMS is delayed or if you are transporting the person a long distance:
   - Use the RICE procedure.
   - Use a splint to stabilize the part against movement.
2. **DO NOT** move or try to straighten an injured extremity (an exception may be made in wilderness or remote locations).
3. Call 9-1-1 for a blue or extremely pale extremity.
4. If bleeding from an open wound is at the injured area:
   - Control bleeding by applying pressure on the wound edges.
   - Cover the exposed bone with a sterile dressing. **DO NOT** push on the bone.

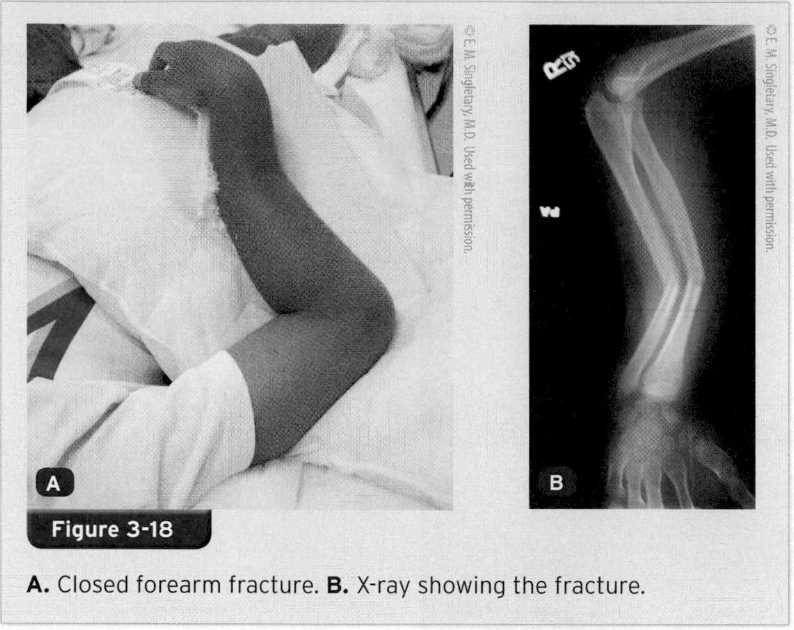

Figure 3-18

A. Closed forearm fracture. **B.** X-ray showing the fracture.

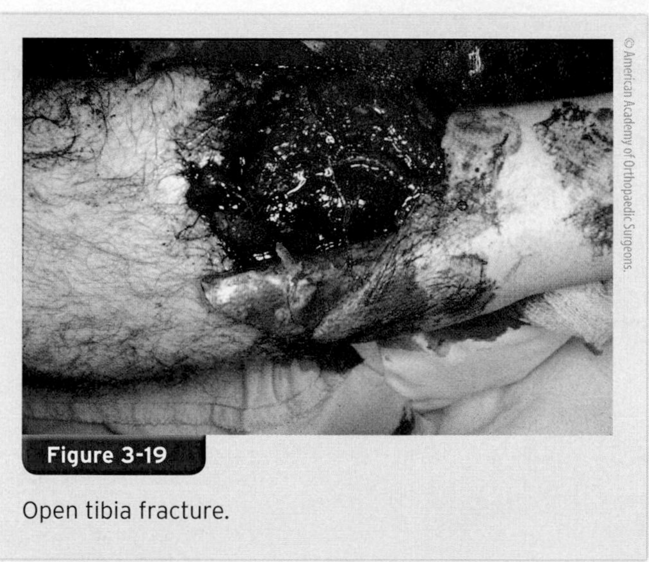

Figure 3-19

Open tibia fracture.

Splinting Guidelines

All broken bones and dislocations should be stabilized before the person is moved. When in doubt, apply a splint. Various objects can be used to stabilize a fracture or dislocation. The device can be rigid (eg, wood board) **Skill Sheet 3-6** or soft (eg, pillow) **Skill Sheet 3-7**. A self-splint

Skill Sheet

3-6 Applying a Rigid Splint on a Forearm

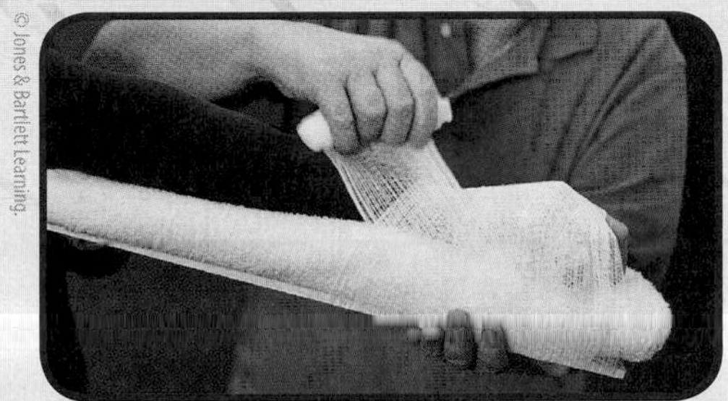

1. Place a rigid object (eg, cardboard, wood board, folded newspaper or magazine) under the forearm. Place padding (eg, towel, T-shirt) between the rigid object and the skin and place padding in the palm (eg, roller bandage, wad of cloth).

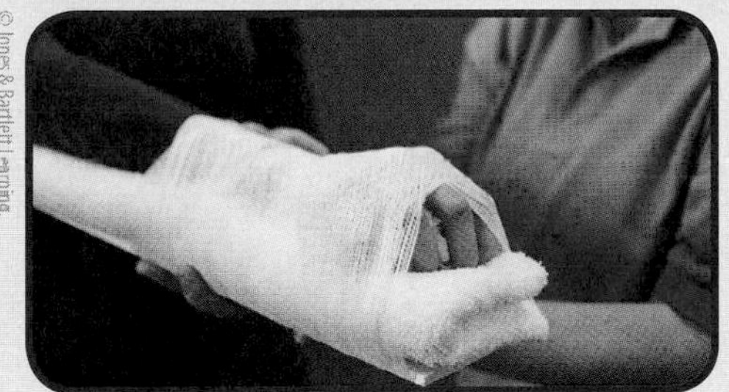

2. Secure the splint onto the arm by using either a roller bandage or folded triangular bandages (known as cravat bandages).

3. Place the arm in a sling with a binder.

Skill Sheet

3-7 Applying a Soft Splint on a Forearm

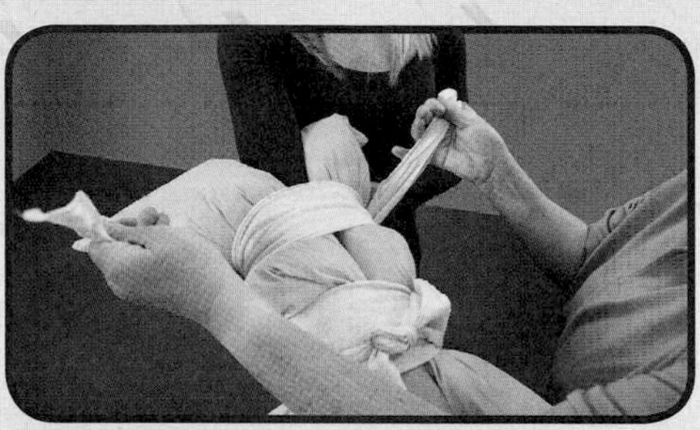

1. Wrap a pillow or folded blanket around the forearm.

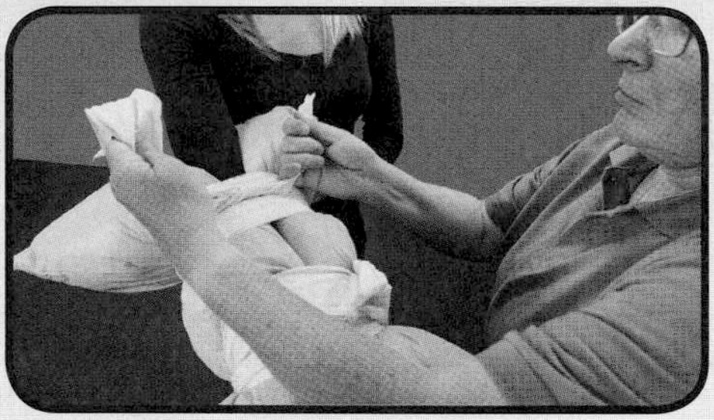

2. Secure the soft splint (eg, pillow) by using folded triangular bandages (known as cravat bandages) or cloth bands.

3. Place the arm in a sling with a binder.

is one in which the injured body part is tied to an uninjured part (eg, injured finger taped to adjacent finger, legs tied together, or arm tied to chest).

1. Cover open wounds with a dry, sterile or clean dressing.
2. Ask the person whether he or she feels you lightly squeezing his or her toes or fingers and ask the person to wiggle his or her toes or fingers unless injured.
3. Apply splints firmly, but not tightly enough to affect blood flow. Pad splints with clothing or other material for comfort. (A broken arm, in addition to being splinted, should be placed in an arm sling and binder Skill Sheet 3-8.)
4. **DO NOT** attempt to replace a dislocated joint.
5. **DO NOT** move a person with a suspected spinal injury unless absolutely necessary.

Skill Sheet

3-8 Applying an Arm Sling

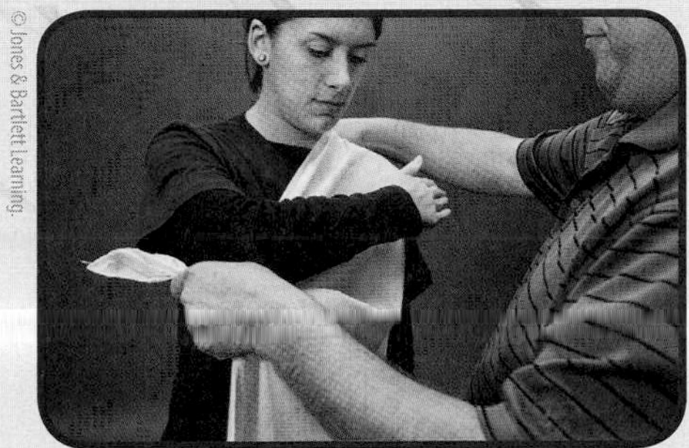

1. Place a triangular bandage between the forearm and chest with the point of the bandage toward the elbow of the injured arm and stretching beyond the elbow. Pull the upper end of the bandage over the uninjured shoulder. Bring the lower end of the bandage over the forearm.

2. Bring the end of the bandage around the neck to the uninjured side and tie to the other end at the hollow above the collar bone (clavicle) on the uninjured side.

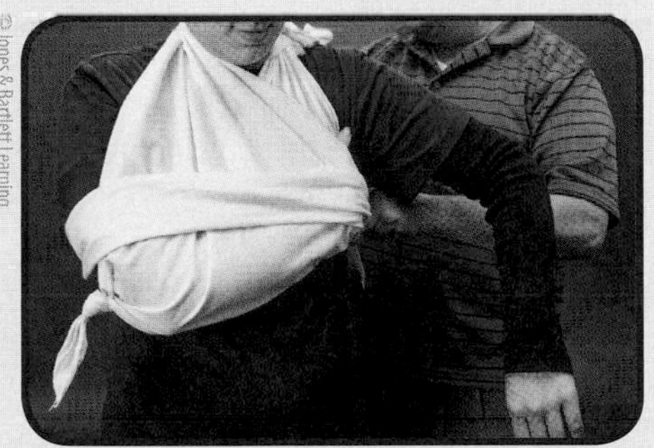

3. If possible, secure the point of the bandage at the elbow with a safety pin or twist it into a pigtail, which can be tied into a knot or tucked inside the sling. Place a binder around the upper arm and body. The center of the binder should be placed over the arm. The hand should be in thumb-up position within the sling and slightly above the level of the elbow. Place padding underneath the knot on the neck for comfort. Adjust the sling to support the hand and wrist; only the fingers should be exposed.

Joint Injuries

A dislocation happens when a joint (eg, shoulder) comes apart and stays apart. Although the injury may not require calling 9-1-1, most people will require medical care. Joint deformity is usually obvious, but it is often difficult to distinguish a dislocation from a severe fracture. Relocation should not be attempted.

What to Look For	What to Do

Dislocation
• Anterior shoulder (accounts for 95% of all shoulder dislocations) Figure 3-20
  • Inability to touch opposite shoulder with the hand of the injured arm
  • Arm is held away from the body
  • Deformity compared to opposite shoulder
  • Extreme pain
• Patella (knee cap) Figure 3-21
  • The knee cap has moved to the outside of the knee joint (large bulge seen under the skin)
  • Deformity compared with opposite knee cap
  • Extreme pain
• Finger Figure 3-22
  • Deformity compared with the finger on the opposite hand
  • Inability to use
	1. Call 9-1-1.
	2. Hold the part when transporting a short distance to a medical facility or until EMS arrives. If EMS is delayed or if you are transporting the person a long distance:
	  • Use the RICE procedure.
	  • Use a splint to stabilize the part against movement.
	3. **DO NOT** try to reduce or reset a dislocation. You may learn in a wilderness first aid course that the following three dislocations may be reset: anterior shoulder, knee cap, and fingers.
	4. If bleeding from an open wound is at the injured area:
	  • Control bleeding by applying pressure on the wound edges.
	  • **DO NOT** push on the bone.

• Sprain Figure 3-23
  • Tenderness/pain
  • Swelling
  • Bruising
	1. Most sprains do not require medical care. If recuperation seems long, consult a physician.
	2. Use the RICE procedure Figure 3-24.

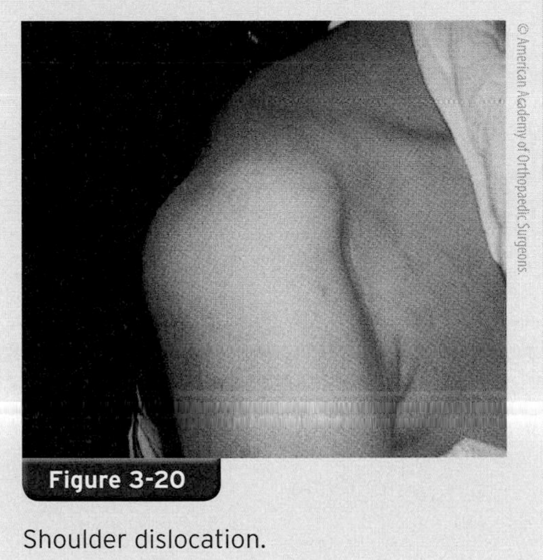

Figure 3-20

Shoulder dislocation.

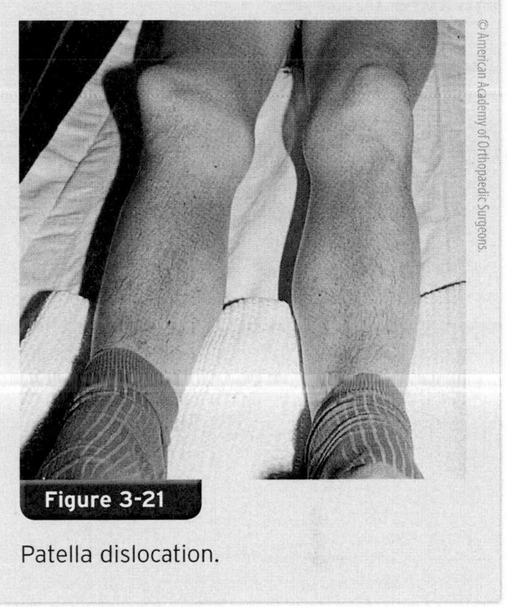

Figure 3-21

Patella dislocation.

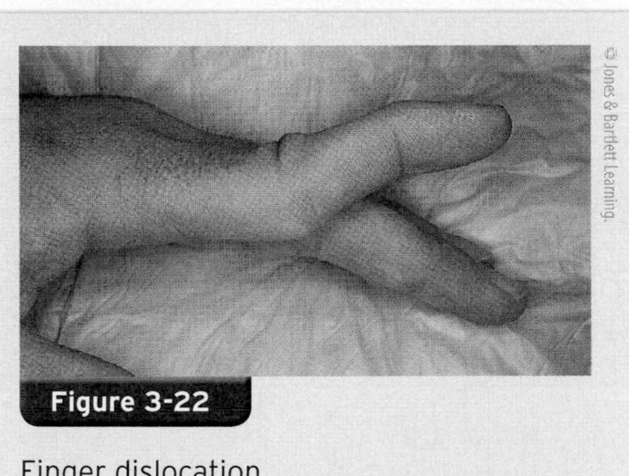

Figure 3-22

Finger dislocation.

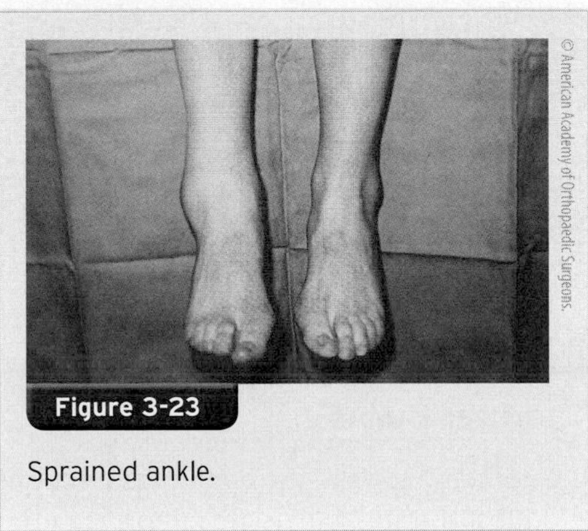

Figure 3-23

Sprained ankle.

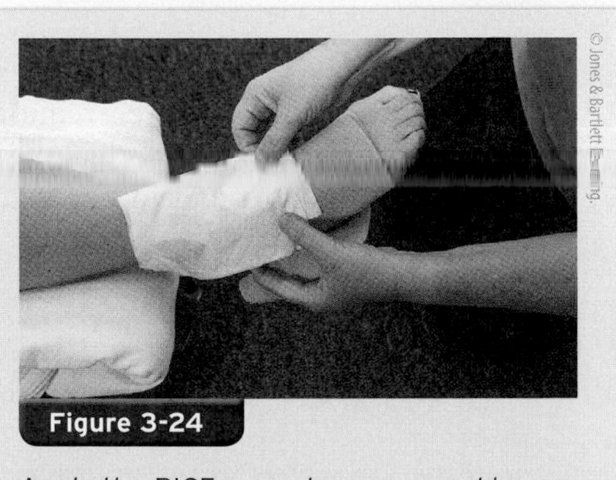

Figure 3-24

Apply the RICE procedure on an ankle sprain, placing a thin cloth or paper towel between the ice pack and skin.

Muscle Injuries

What to Look For	What to Do
• Sudden muscle pain • A muscle, often the calf muscle, that feels hard because of muscle contraction • Residual discomfort, which may last for a few hours	1. Suspect a muscle cramp (spasm). 2. Try one or more of these methods to relax the muscle: • Gently stretch the affected muscle. • Press on the muscle. • Apply an ice pack to the muscle. • If cramping occurs during exertion in a hot environment, drink lightly salted cool water (one-fourth teaspoon [1.25 mL] salt in 1 quart [about 1 L] of water) or a commercial sports drink. 3. **DO NOT** give salt tablets.
• Blow to a muscle • Swelling • Tenderness and pain • Black and blue mark appearing hours later	1. Suspect a muscle bruise (contusion). 2. Use the RICE procedure.
• Occurs during physical activity • Sharp pain • Extreme tenderness • Inability to use injured part • Stiffness and pain when muscle is used	1. Suspect muscle strain (pull). 2. Use the RICE procedure.

▶ Burns

Thermal Burns

Before helping, take the appropriate actions described on pages 5–6.

Most thermal burns are minor. Superficial and small partial-thickness burns rarely require medical care. In contrast, medical care is needed as soon as possible for large partial-thickness and all full-thickness burns, burned airways, and circumferential burns (completely around body part):

1. Stop the burning! If clothing is on fire, have the person roll on the ground using the "stop, drop, and roll" method. Smother the flames with a blanket, or douse the person with water. Remove clothing and all jewelry, especially rings, from the burn area.
2. Check and monitor breathing if the person inhaled heated air or was in an explosion.
3. Determine the depth of the burn. This may be difficult but it will help determine what first aid to give.

4. Determine the size of the burn by using the Rule of the Hand. The person's hand (including the palm, closed fingers, and thumb) equals about 1% of his or her body surface area (BSA).
5. Determine which parts of the body are burned. Burns on the face, hands, feet, and genitals are more severe than burns on other body parts.
6. Seek medical care or call 9-1-1 for the following:
   - Burns on the face, neck, hands, feet, or genitals
   - Breathing difficulty
   - Blistering or broken skin
   - Large area burned (ie, back, trunk)
   - All third- and large second-degree burns
   - Other concerns (ie, coughing, wheezing, hoarse voice, or carbon monoxide exposure)

What to Look For	What to Do
First-degree burn (superficial) Figure 3-25, indicated by: • Redness • Mild swelling • Tenderness • Pain	1. Immerse the burned area in cool or cold water, place it under running cold water, or apply a wet, cool or cold compress for at least 10 minutes as soon as possible Figure 3-26. If cold water is unavailable, use any other available cold liquid. **DO NOT** apply ice, ice water, or salt water. 2. Give ibuprofen (for children, give acetaminophen). 3. Have the person drink as much water as possible without becoming nauseous. 4. Keep burned arm or leg raised. 5. After burn has been cooled, apply aloe vera gel or an inexpensive skin moisturizer. First-degree burns do not need to be covered.
Small second-degree burn of less than 20% BSA (partial-thickness) Figure 3-27, indicated by: • Blisters • Swelling • Weeping of fluids • Severe pain	Follow Steps 1 through 4 for first-degree burns, with the following additions: 1. After burn has been cooled, apply thin layer of antibacterial ointment on it. 2. Cover burn with a loose, dry, nonstick, sterile or clean dressing. 3. **DO NOT** break any blisters.
Large second-degree burn of more than 20% BSA (partial-thickness)	Follow Steps 1 through 4 for first-degree burns, with the following additions: 1. Apply cold, but monitor, as it may cause hypothermia. 2. Call 9-1-1.

(continued)

What to Look For	What to Do
Third-degree burn (full-thickness) Figure 3-28, indicated by: • Dry, leathery, gray colored, or charred skin	1. Cover burn with a dry, nonstick, sterile or clean dressing. 2. Call 9-1-1.

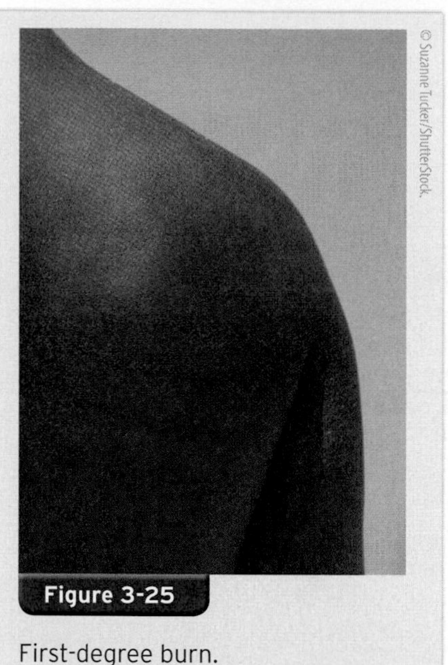

Figure 3-25

First-degree burn.

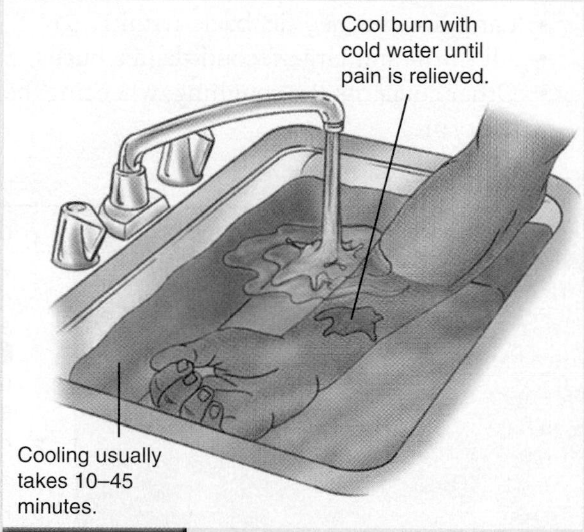

Figure 3-26

Run the burned area under water to cool the burn.

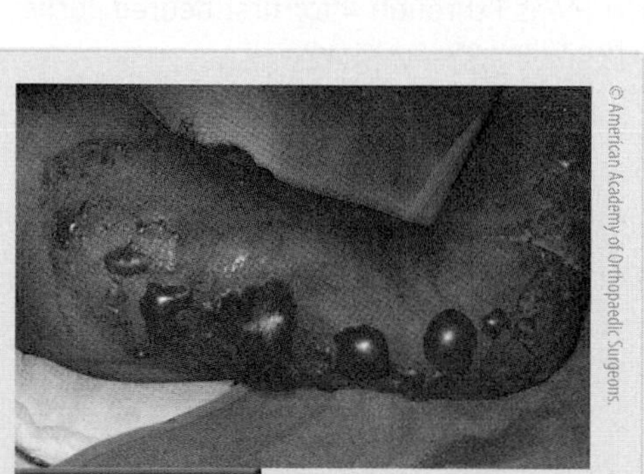

Figure 3-27

Second-degree burn.

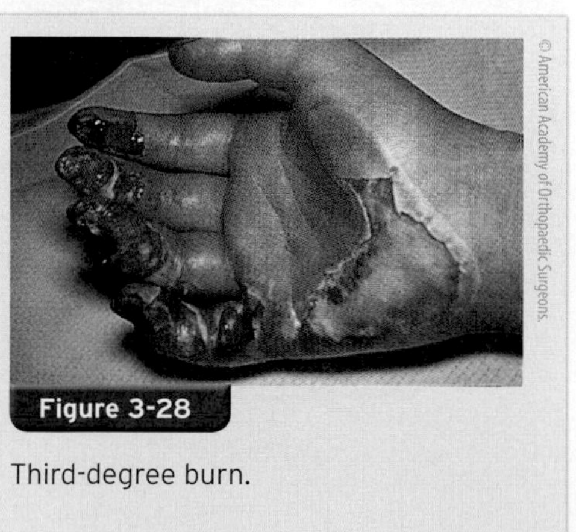

Figure 3-28

Third-degree burn.

Electrical Burns

Before helping, take the appropriate actions described on pages 5–6.

Every person who has been electrocuted needs medical care; 9-1-1 must be called. The major damage occurs inside the body; therefore, the outside burn might appear small **Figure 3-29**. If the person is inside a building and still in contact with electricity (power cord, electrical device, bare wire), turn off the electricity at the fuse box, circuit breaker, or outside switch box, or unplug the appliance. If the electrocuted person is in contact with a high-tension power line, take the following steps:

- Call 9-1-1 to have the electricity turned off or wires cut.
- **DO NOT** touch or move the power lines or person.
- **DO NOT** try to move electrical wires or devices with a wooden pole, rope, or any other item.
- Keep people away from the area.

What to Look For	What to Do
• Burn wound, which might appear small • Entrance and exit wounds (Usually, the electricity exits where the body is touching a surface or is in contact with a ground [ie, a metal object]; this is often the hand or foot.) • Multiple burns (Most electrical burns are third-degree burns.) • Absent breathing/pulse (Electricity can cause a person's breathing or heart to stop.)	Once the area is safe: 1. Check breathing and, if absent, begin CPR. 2. Call 9-1-1 immediately. Every person who has been electrocuted needs medical care. 3. If the person fell, check for broken bones and a spinal injury. 4. Most electrical burns are third-degree burns, so cover all burn wounds with sterile dressings.

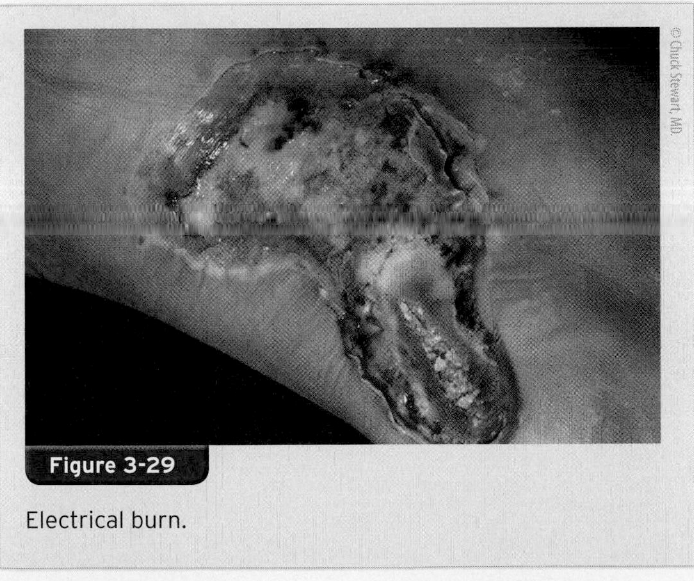

Figure 3-29

Electrical burn.

Chemical Burns

Before helping, take the appropriate actions described on pages 5–6.

Avoid chemical contact; wear gloves and, if available, goggles Figure 3-30. If the burn occurred at a workplace, send someone to check the safety data sheets (SDSs) for the hazardous materials used at the worksite. SDSs include first aid procedures. The Occupational Safety and Health Administration requires employers to identify chemical hazards using labels Figure 3-31.

What to Look For	What to Do
• Pain • Burning • Breathing difficulty • Eye pain or vision changes	First aid is the same for most chemical burns. Once the area is safe: 1. Brush a dry or powder chemical off the skin with a gloved hand or piece of cloth before flushing with water. 2. Flush the burn immediately with large amounts of cool running water for at least 20 minutes or until EMS arrives. Clothing can be removed while flushing. 3. Call 9-1-1 immediately for all chemical burns. 4. **DO NOT** try to neutralize the chemical. 5. For a chemical in an eye: Tip the head so the affected eye is below the nose, and wash the eye with warm water (which is tolerated in the eye better than cold water) from nose out to side of face for at least 20 minutes.

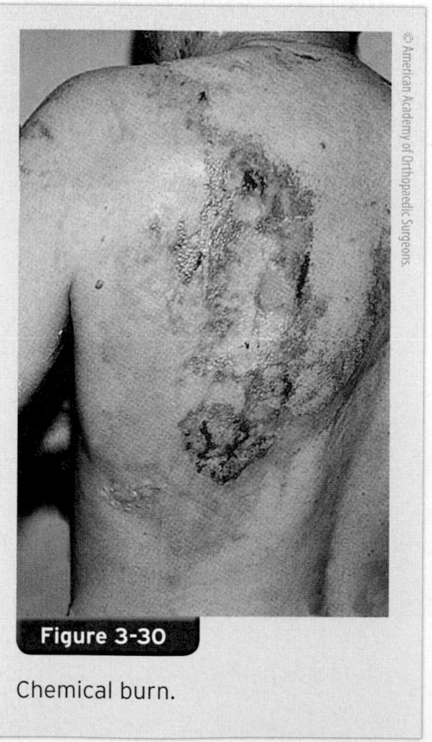

Figure 3-30

Chemical burn.

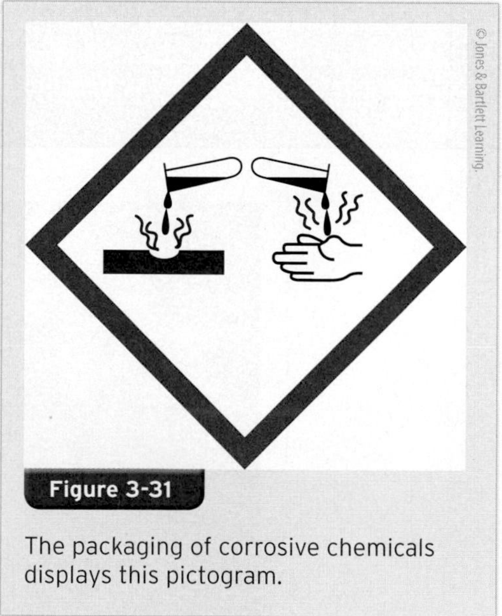

Figure 3-31

The packaging of corrosive chemicals displays this pictogram.

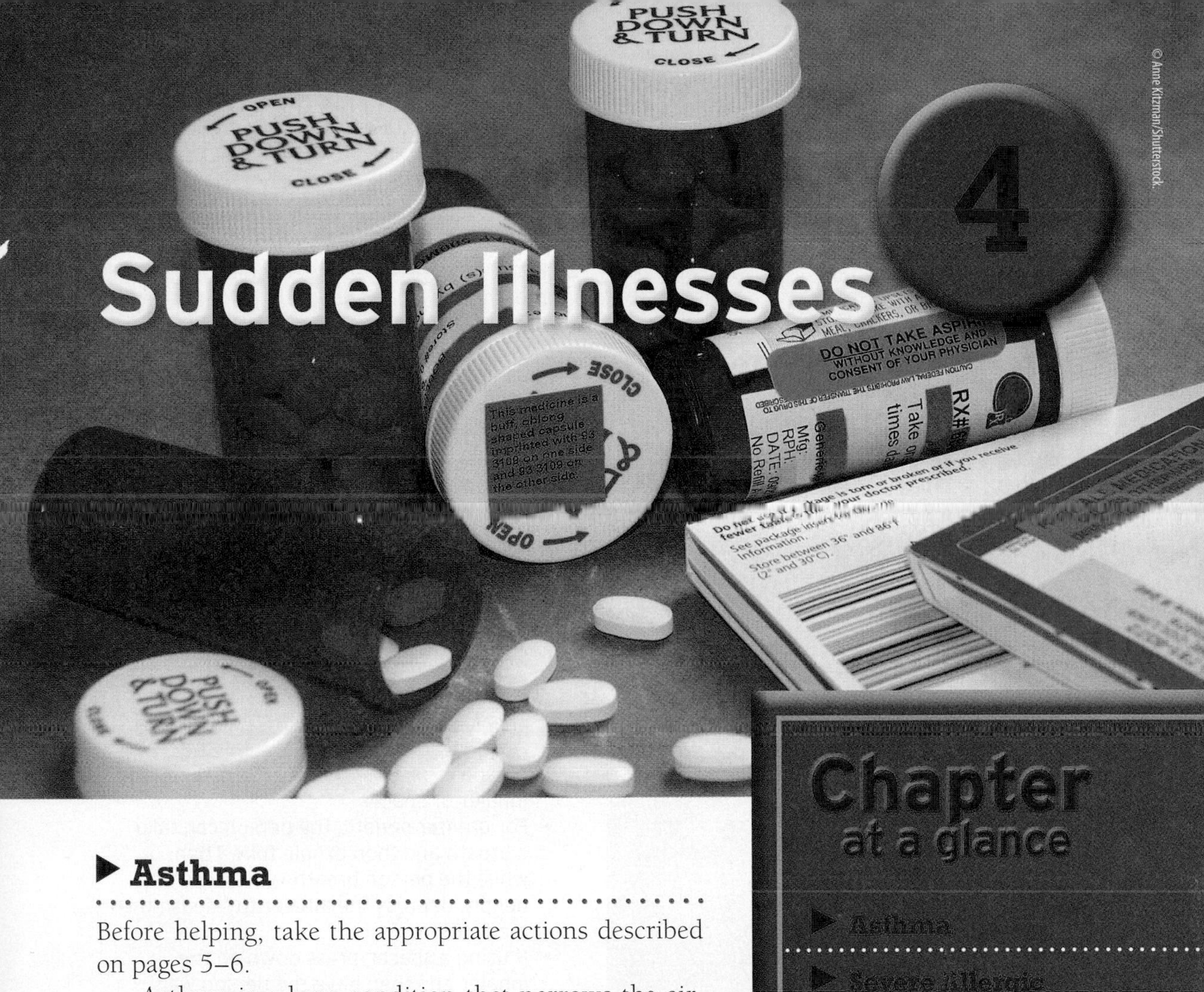

4 Sudden Illnesses

Chapter at a glance

▶ Asthma

Before helping, take the appropriate actions described on pages 5–6.

Asthma is a lung condition that narrows the airway (the tubes that carry air into and out of the lungs). Episodes can occur occasionally or often. Between episodes, the person has no trouble breathing. Asthma varies from one person to another, with symptoms ranging from mild to severe, and can be life threatening.

What to Look For

- Frequent coughing
- Wheezing-high-pitched whistling sound or squeaky sound during breathing
- Chest tightness
- Shortness of breath
- Sitting in tripod position (leaning forward with hands on knees or other support, trying to breathe)
- Inability to speak in complete sentences without stopping to breathe
- Nostrils flaring with each breath
- Fast breath and heart rates
- Blue lips or fingernails

What to Do

1. Place the person in an upright sitting position, leaning slightly forward.
2. Encourage the person to sit quietly and breathe slowly and deeply in through the nose and out through the mouth.
3. Call 9-1-1 immediately if the person is struggling to breathe, talk, or stay awake; has blue lips or fingernails; has no medicine; or asks for an ambulance.
4. Ask the person about any asthma medication he or she uses. Most people with asthma have a physician-prescribed quick-relief (rescue) inhaler with a spacer or holding chamber **Figure 4-1**.
5. Help the person use his or her quick-relief inhaler:
   - Shake the inhaler vigorously several times, remove the cap, and apply the spacer if available **Figure 4-2**.
   - Holding the inhaler upright, tell the person to place his or her lips around the inhaler or spacer.
   - For greater benefit, the person can take a breath and then exhale fully. Then, while the person breathes in slowly and deeply, depress the inhaler to release the medication.
   - If using a spacer, press down on the inhaler and then have the person wait 5 seconds before breathing in.
   - Tell the person to hold his or her breath for at least 10 seconds and to breathe out slowly.
   - A second dose may be given in 30 to 60 seconds.
6. Call 9-1-1 if:
   - There is no improvement after using the medication.
   - Repeated attacks occur.
   - A severe and prolonged attack occurs.

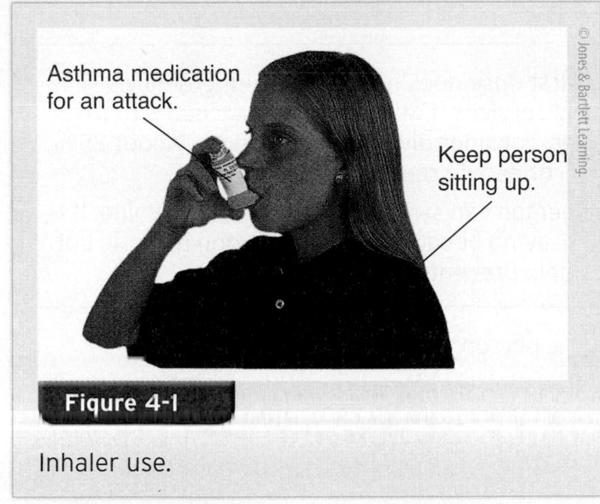

Figure 4-1

Inhaler use.

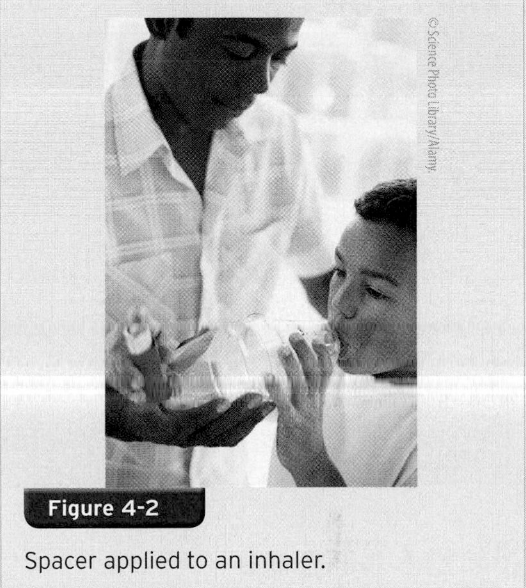

Figure 4-2

Spacer applied to an inhaler.

▶ Severe Allergic Reactions (Anaphylaxis)

Before helping, take the appropriate actions described on pages 5–6.

Severe reactions to medications, food and food additives, and insect stings (called anaphylaxis) can be life threatening.

What to Look For	What to Do
Severe allergic reaction (anaphylaxis), indicated by: • Shortness of breath • Swelling of tongue, mouth, nose • Intense itching • Flushed skin or swollen face • Sneezing, coughing, wheezing • Tightness and swelling in the throat • Tightness in the chest • Increased heart rate • Blueness around lips and mouth • Dizziness • Nausea and vomiting • Reports from the person of having previous severe allergic reactions • Medical identification tag	1. Call 9-1-1. 2. Monitor breathing. 3. If the person has his or her own physician-prescribed epinephrine auto-injector, you may need to get it and help the person self-administer it **Figure 4-3**. If the person is not capable of using it and you are allowed by state law to give an injection, use the person's prescribed epinephrine auto-injector **Skill Sheet 4-1**. • Find the injection site on the outer midthigh between the knee and the hip. Check for coins, keys, and pant seams, which could obstruct the needle. • Remove the safety cap. • Push the auto-injector until you hear a click against the outer midthigh (if necessary, the injection can be done through light clothing). • Hold in place for 10 seconds. • Pull the auto-injector straight out from the leg. • Rub the area for 10 seconds.

(continued)

What to Look For	What to Do
	4. If the first dose does not help and emergency medical services (EMS) arrival will exceed 5 to 10 minutes, consider giving a second dose. About 25% to 35% of people require a second dose. 5. If the person can swallow, give an antihistamine. It is not lifesaving because it takes too long to work, but it can help prevent further reactions.
Mild allergic reaction, indicated by: • Red, itchy eyes • Itchy, sneezing, runny nose • Rash on skin, usually on one part of body	1. Help the person: • Self-administer his or her asthma rescue inhaler, and/or • Take an antihistamine.

Skill Sheet

4-1 Using an Epinephrine Auto-Injector

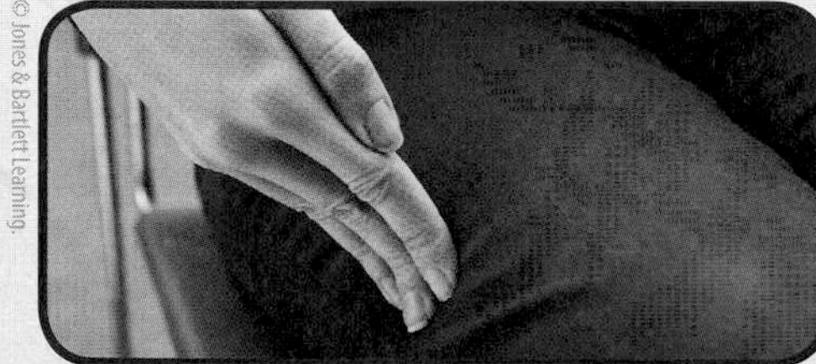

1. Find the injection site on the side of the person's thigh, halfway between the knee and the hip. Check for coins, keys, and pant seams, which could obstruct the needle.

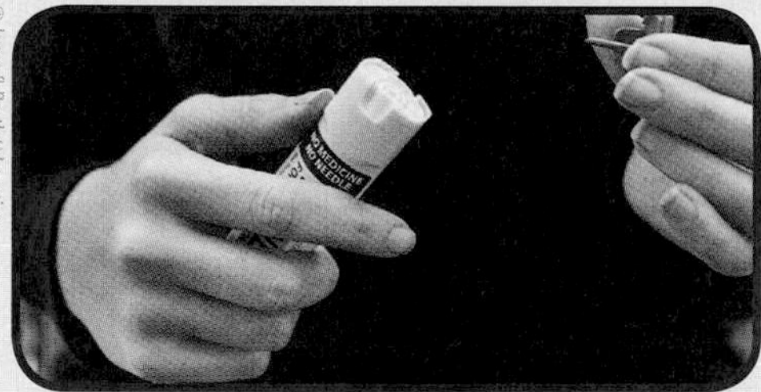

2. Take off the safety cap of the epinephrine auto-injector.

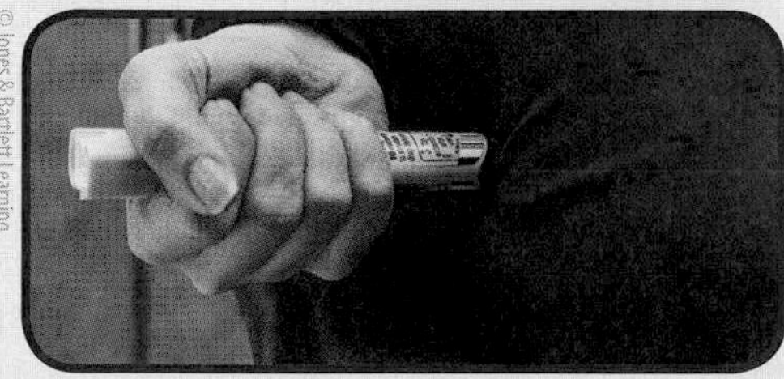

3. Hold the epinephrine auto-injector without touching either end of the pen. Push the auto-injector firmly against the thigh until you hear a click. Hold in place for about 10 sec. Pull the auto-injector straight out from the leg. Rub the injection site for about 10 sec.

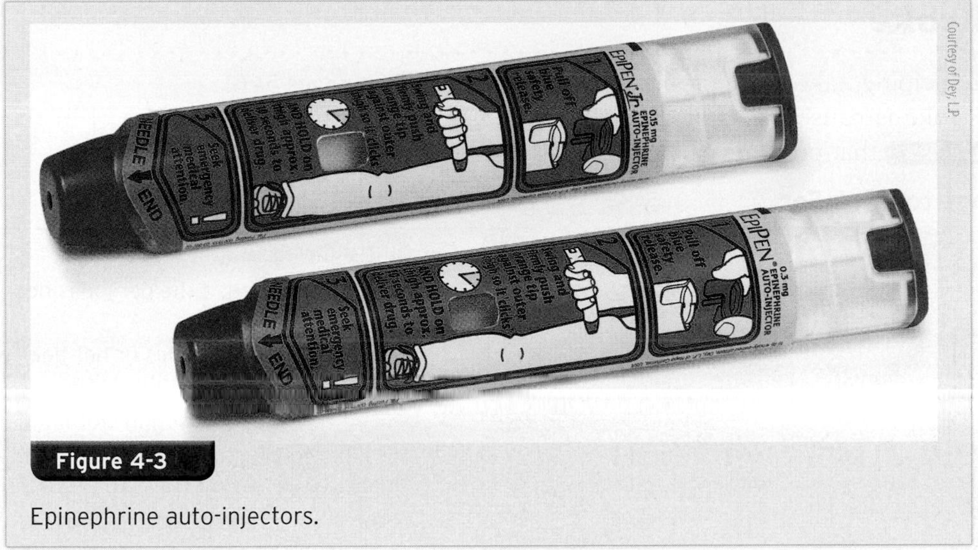

Courtesy of Dey, L.P.

Figure 4-3

Epinephrine auto-injectors.

▶ Heart Attack

Before helping, take the appropriate actions described on pages 5–6.

In a heart attack, the heart muscle tissue dies because its blood supply has been severely reduced or stopped. Heart attacks can be difficult to determine. Thirty-five percent of people who sustain a heart attack never experience chest pain.

What to Look For

- Chest pain that feels like pressure, squeezing, or fullness, usually in the center of the chest. It may also be felt in the jaw, shoulder, arms, or back; back or jaw pain is more common in women. The pain may last for more than 5 minutes, or it may come and go.
- Sweating or cold sweats
- Light-headedness or dizziness
- Nausea or vomiting (more common in women)
- Numbness, aching, or tingling in the arm (usually the left arm)
- Shortness of breath (more common in women)
- Weakness or fatigue, especially in older adults

What to Do

1. Have the person sit, with knees raised, and lean against a stable support (eg, wall, fence post, tree trunk). Try to keep the person calm. **DO NOT** allow the person to walk.
2. Call 9-1-1 immediately. **DO NOT** drive the person to a medical facility; wait for EMS to arrive.
3. While waiting for EMS to arrive:
   - Loosen any tight clothing.
   - Ask if the person takes any chest pain medication, such as nitroglycerin, for a known heart condition, and, if so, help him or her take it.
   - If the person is alert, is able to swallow, is not allergic to aspirin, and has no signs of stroke, help the person take one adult aspirin (325 mg) or two to four low-dose baby aspirins (81 mg each). Pulverize or have the person crunch them with his or her teeth before swallowing for faster results.
   - Monitor breathing. If the person becomes unresponsive and stops breathing, begin cardiopulmonary resuscitation (CPR).

Stroke

Before helping, take the appropriate actions described on pages 5–6.

Stroke is caused by a blockage **Figure 4-4** or rupture of a blood vessel in the brain **Figure 4-5** that prevents part of the brain from getting the blood flow it needs.

What to Look For	What to Do
The acronym **FAST** acts as an assessment tool to be used to determine if a stroke may have occurred: • **F**ace: Ask the person to smile. It is abnormal to have one side of the face not move well compared with the other side. • **A**rms: Ask the person to close his or her eyes and raise both arms with the palms up. It is abnormal if one arm drifts downward when held extended. • **S**peech: Ask the person to repeat a simple phrase (eg, "The sky is blue."). It is abnormal if the person slurs words, uses the wrong words, or cannot speak at all. • **T**ime: Seek medical help if any of the signs discussed earlier occur. The presence of one of these signs is associated with a high risk of stroke (72%); if all three are present, the risk is as high as 85%.	Call 9-1-1 and while waiting for EMS: 1. Monitor breathing. If the person is not breathing, begin CPR. 2. Position the person on his or her back with head and shoulders slightly raised. 3. Loosen tight or constricting clothing. 4. Be prepared to turn the person onto his or her side to allow drool or vomit to drain. 5. If the person is unresponsive but breathing, place on his or her side.

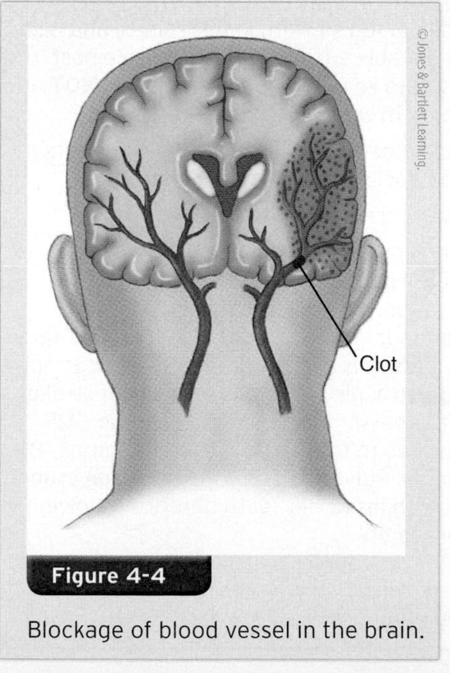

Figure 4-4

Blockage of blood vessel in the brain.

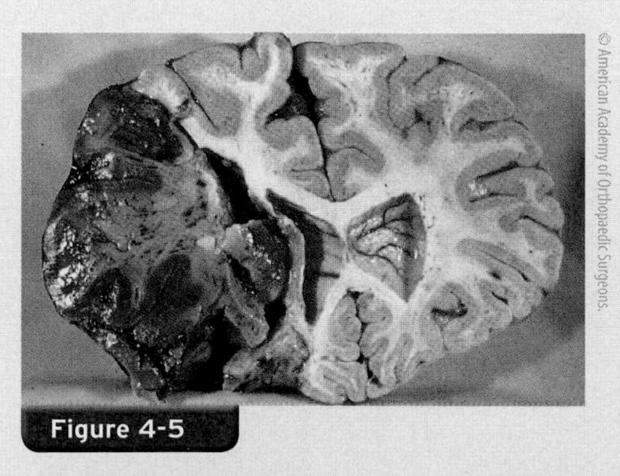

Figure 4-5

Rupture of blood vessel in the brain.

▶ Fainting

Before helping, take the appropriate actions described on pages 5–6.

What to Look For	What to Do
• A person that has suddenly collapsed • Pale skin, lips, and nail beds • Clammy, sweaty skin	1. Check breathing. 2. If breathing has stopped, call 9-1-1 and give CPR. 3. If the person is breathing: • Keep the person flat on his or her back. Feet can be raised 6 to 12 inches (15 to 30 cm) if it does not cause pain. • Monitor breathing; if it stops, give CPR. • Loosen tight clothing. • If the person fell, check and treat any injuries. • Wipe the person's forehead with a cool, wet cloth. • **DO NOT** use ammonia inhalants or smelling salts. • **DO NOT** give the person anything to drink or eat until he or she has fully recovered and can swallow. • **DO NOT** splash or pour water on the person's face. • **DO NOT** slap the person's face in an attempt to revive him or her. 4. Seek medical care if: • There are repeated episodes. • The person fainted for no apparent reason. • The person does not regain responsiveness quickly. • The person has diabetes, has seizures, is pregnant, has a loss of bowel or bladder control, or is over age 50.
A person that is about to faint	1. Prevent a hard fall if possible. 2. If the person collapses, take the steps discussed earlier.

▶ Diabetic Emergencies

Before helping, take the appropriate actions described on pages 5–6.

Most people with diabetes monitor their blood glucose levels as often as four times a day to maintain the proper levels and to prevent a diabetic emergency Figure 4-6. "Sugar (glucose) for everyone" is the rule of thumb for all diabetic emergencies.

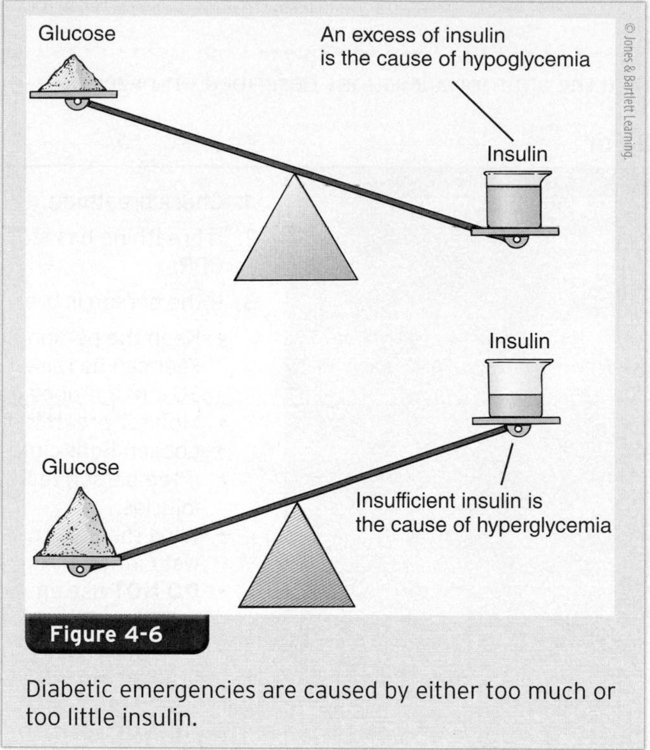

Figure 4-6

Diabetic emergencies are caused by either too much or too little insulin.

Hypoglycemia (Blood Glucose Too Low)

Hypoglycemia is a life-threatening emergency that occurs when a person with diabetes does one of the following:

- Takes too much insulin (rapidly depletes sugar)
- Does not eat (reduces sugar intake)
- Overexerts self or exercises (uses sugar faster)
- Vomits (empties stomach of sugar)

What to Look For	What to Do
• Responsive, alert, and can swallow • Medical identification tag • Sudden onset of symptoms (minutes to an hour) because no sugar is reaching the brain • Staggering, poor coordination, clumsiness	The person may be able to tell you what to do. 1. If the person has a blood glucose monitor, allow him or her to check blood glucose. 2. Use the Rule of 15 when: • Testing is not possible. • Testing shows a low blood glucose level. • Profuse sweating or shaking occurs in a person with diabetes.

What to Look For	What to Do
• Anger, bad temper • Cold, pale, moist, or clammy skin • Confusion, disorientation • Sudden hunger • Excessive sweating • Trembling, shakiness	The Rule of 15 works as follows: • Have the person eat 15 grams of sugar (ie, 3 to 5 glucose tablets, 3 to 5 teaspoons [15 mL to 25 mL] of table sugar, or 4 ounces [118 mL] of orange juice or regular soft drink [not diet]) Figure 4-7. • Wait 15 minutes for the sugar to get into the blood. • Recheck the blood glucose level. If it is still low or no testing is available, give the person 15 more grams of sugar to consume Figure 4-8. **3.** If there is still no improvement, call 9-1-1 as soon as possible.
• Unresponsive • Unable to follow simple instructions • Has seizures • Unable to swallow	**1.** Call 9-1-1 immediately. **2.** Monitor breathing. **3.** Look for a medical identification tag. **4.** **DO NOT** give any food or drink. **5.** Place the person on his or her side to keep the airway open and to drain fluids or vomit from the mouth.

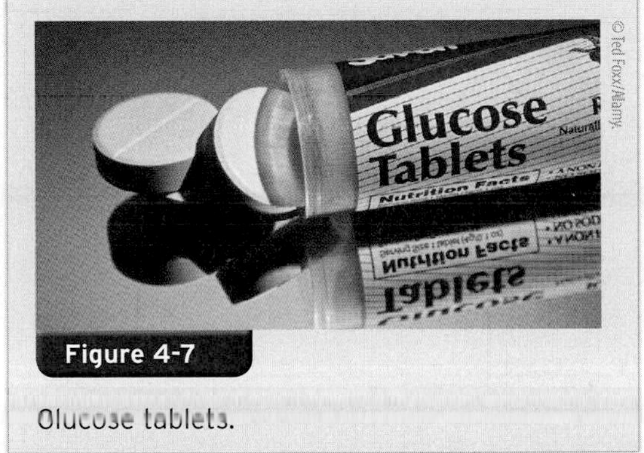

© Ted Foxx/Alamy.

Figure 4-7

Glucose tablets.

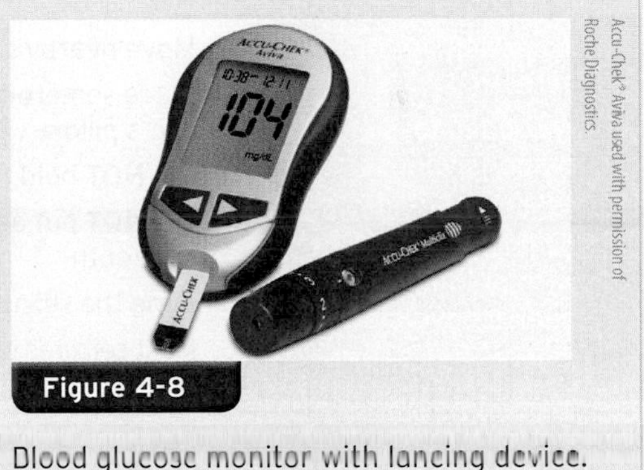

Accu-Chek® Aviva used with permission of Roche Diagnostics.

Figure 4-8

Blood glucose monitor with lancing device.

Hyperglycemia (Blood Glucose Too High)

Hyperglycemia occurs when a person with diabetes has too much sugar in his or her blood. Several conditions can cause hyperglycemia (ie, insufficient insulin, overeating, illness, inactivity, stress, or a combination of these factors). Most people with diabetes can recognize what is happening and will adjust their insulin dose or seek medical help before serious problems develop; however, if it is not treated within 24 hours, hyperglycemia can be fatal.

What to Look For	What to Do
• Medical identification tag • Gradual onset (hours to days) because some sugar is still reaching the brain • Drowsiness • Extreme thirst • Very frequent urination • Warm, red, dry skin • Vomiting • Fruity breath odor (has also been described to be like nail polish remover) • Heavy breathing • Eventual unresponsiveness	1. Give frequent, small sips of water if the person with diabetes can swallow. 2. If uncertain whether the person with diabetes has a high or low blood glucose level, and if he or she is responsive and able to swallow, use the Rule of 15 for giving sugar, as previously described. The extra sugar will not cause significant harm in a person experiencing hyperglycemia. 3. **DO NOT** give insulin unless the person with diabetes can self-administer it. 4. Call 9-1-1 as soon as possible.

Seizures

Before helping, take the appropriate actions described on pages 5–6.

Seizures result from a disturbance of the electrical activity in the brain, causing uncontrollable muscle movements. Causes include epilepsy, head injury, brain tumor, stroke, heat stroke, poisoning (including alcohol or drugs), diabetic emergency, and high fever.

What to Look For	What to Do
• A sudden cry or scream • A sudden loss of responsiveness • Rigid body followed by jerky movement with arching of the back (convulsions) • Foaming at mouth • Drooling from mouth • Grinding of teeth • Blue face and lips • Eyes rolling upward • Loss of bladder or bowel control	1. Move nearby objects to avoid injury. 2. Place something soft under the head such as a rolled towel. **DO NOT** use a pillow. 3. **DO NOT** hold the person down. 4. **DO NOT** put anything between the person's teeth or give anything by mouth. 5. Time the seizure from start to finish. 6. Most seizures do not require medical care and end in 1 to 2 minutes. 7. Keep bystanders away. 8. Call 9-1-1 for any of the following: • Seizure lasting longer than 5 minutes • Series of seizures following one another • The person has breathing difficulties after the seizure • The person has diabetes or is pregnant • Seizure happened in water • This is the person's first known seizure • The seizure is injury-related • Slow recovery

What to Look For	What to Do
	9. After the seizure: • Keep the airway open by placing the person on his or her side and head on a rolled towel. • Monitor breathing and if it stops, give CPR. • Allow the person to sleep. • Stay with the person until he or she is alert.

▶ Shock

Before helping, take the appropriate actions described on pages 5–6.

Shock happens when the body tissues do not get enough oxygen-rich blood. Do not confuse this condition with an electrical shock or "being shocked," as in scared or surprised. Shock is life threatening. Expect and treat for shock if a person has any of the following conditions:

- Massive external or internal bleeding
- A severe infection
- Multiple severe broken bones
- Sign of a heart attack
- Abdominal or chest injury
- Severe allergic reaction

Even if there are no signs of shock, you should still follow the procedures for injured people found in the following table.

What to Look For	What to Do
• Altered mental status (anxiety and restlessness) • Pale, cold, and clammy skin, lips, and nail beds • Nausea/vomiting • Rapid breathing and heart rate • Unresponsiveness when shock is severe	1. Treat injuries. 2. If responsive and breathing normally, keep the person flat on his or her back. If there is no sign of injury (ie, fainting, dehydration, non-injury bleeding), another option is to raise the feet 6 to 12 inches (15 to 30 cm), if it does not cause pain **Figure 4-9**. 3. If unresponsive, roll the person onto his or her side. 4. Prevent the loss of body heat by putting blankets or coats under and over the person. 5. If the person does not improve, call 9-1-1. 6. **DO NOT** give anything to eat or drink unless medical help is delayed over 1 hour, in which case, sips of water can be given if fluids do not cause nausea and/or vomiting.

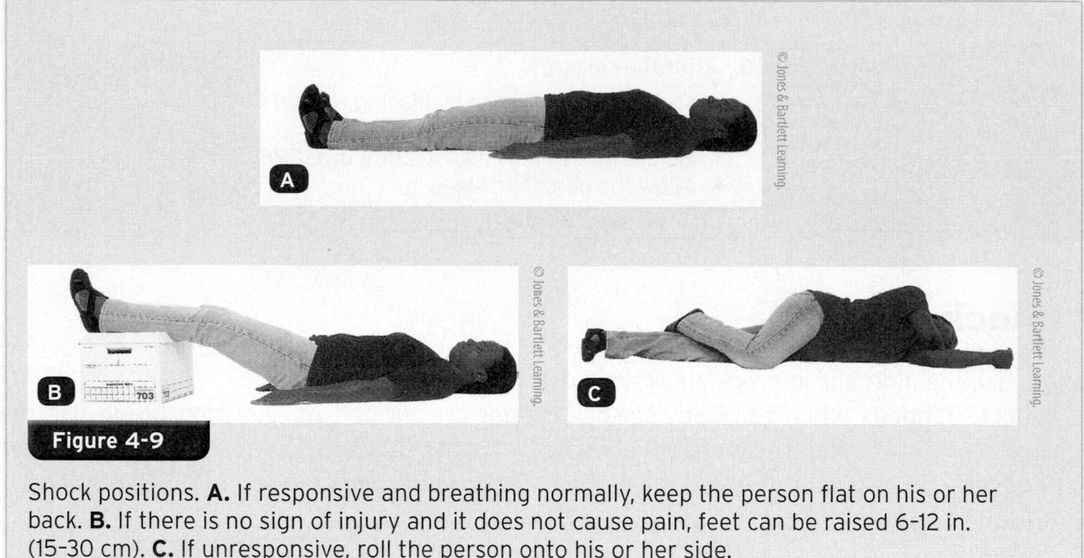

Figure 4-9

Shock positions. **A.** If responsive and breathing normally, keep the person flat on his or her back. **B.** If there is no sign of injury and it does not cause pain, feet can be raised 6-12 in. (15-30 cm). **C.** If unresponsive, roll the person onto his or her side.

▶ Pregnancy Complications

Before helping, take the appropriate actions described on pages 5–6.

Ask the woman if she might be pregnant.

What to Look For	What to Do
Severe stomach pain or cramps (Short, mild cramps near the delivery date may be normal; the woman may be in labor if cramps are strong and repeat, or her water has broken.)	If pain persists or labor is suspected, seek immediate medical care.
Seizure (may indicate a serious complication)	1. Provide appropriate care for seizures. (See pages 64-65). 2. Call 9-1-1 immediately.
Vaginal bleeding	1. Have the woman place a sanitary pad or a towel to absorb blood. **DO NOT** pack the vagina. 2. Call 9-1-1 immediately.
Sudden leakage of fluid (may indicate the beginning of labor)	Seek immediate medical care.
Morning sickness	1. Treat the vomiting. 2. If vomiting persists, seek medical care.

Environmental Emergencies

5

Chapter at a glance

▶ Animal Bites

Before helping, take the appropriate actions described on pages 5–6.

For bites from an animal, notify the animal's owner, or, if you are the owner, notify the family of the person who was bitten **Figure 5-1**. When doing so, use good judgment because encounters may become very emotional and lead to violence. If the bite came from a wild animal, notify the proper authorities.

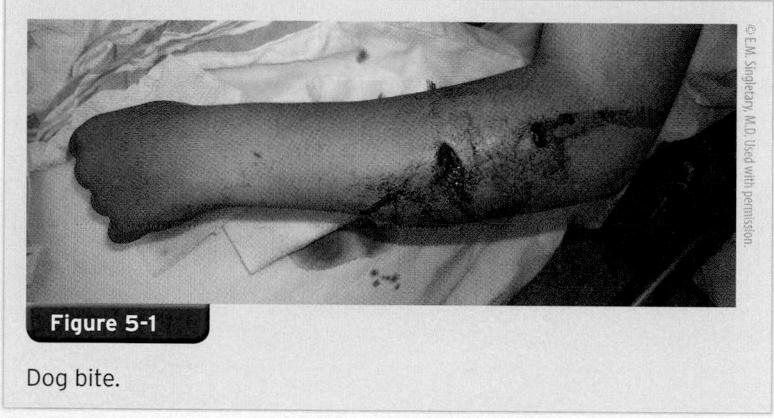

Figure 5-1

Dog bite.

What to Look For	What to Do
Bite that has broken the skin	1. Stop the bleeding by applying direct pressure over the wound. 2. For a shallow wound: • Wash inside and around it with soap and running water. • Flush the inside of the wound with clean running water. • Cover the wound with a thin layer of an over-the-counter (OTC) antibiotic ointment and a sterile dressing. 3. Severe bites should be cleaned at a medical facility. 4. For all bites that break the skin, seek medical care to: • Clean the wound. • Close wide and gaping open wounds. • Receive a tetanus booster, if necessary.
Bite that did not break the skin	Apply an ice pack to the skin for up to 20 minutes.
Wild animal bite	1. **DO NOT** try to capture the animal. 2. **DO NOT** kill the animal. If you must kill it, **DO NOT** hit or shoot its head (brain). Though often impossible, the animal's brain can be tested for the rabies virus. 3. Contact the local health department.

▶ Snake and Other Reptile Bites

Before helping, take the appropriate actions described on pages 5–6.

In about 25% of venomous snakebites, venom is not injected—only fang and tooth wounds (known as a dry bite) occur. Never assume, however, that the bite is a dry bite. Take the following steps if you see fang marks and positively identify a pit viper:

- Get the person and bystanders away from the snake because of the risk of a second bite. A dead snake can still bite even if decapitated.
- Encourage the person to rest, stay calm, and be still.
- **DO NOT** try to capture or kill the snake. These actions could lead to a second person being bitten. Try to remember the snake's color and the shape of its head. Taking a good photograph from a safe distance (more than the length of the snake) can help with identifying the snake.

- Remove any rings, jewelry, or tight clothing from the bitten body part to avoid constriction from swelling.
- Gently wash the bite with soap and running water and apply a sterile dressing over the fang marks.
- Call 9-1-1 or transport the person to a medical facility as soon as possible.

Reptile	What to Look For	What to Do
Pit Vipers Include: • Rattlesnakes Figure 5-2 • Copperheads Figure 5-3 • Cottonmouths/ water moccasins Figure 5-4 Identified by: • Triangular, flat head, wider than the neck • Vertical, elliptical pupils (cat's eye) • Heat-sensitive pit located between the eye and nostril • Only rattlesnakes have rattles on their tails.	• Severe, burning pain at the bite site • Two small puncture wounds (the person may have only one) Figure 5-5 • Swelling within 10 to 15 minutes; may involve entire extremity • Discoloration and blood-filled blisters possible in 6 to 10 hours • Nausea, vomiting, sweating, and weakness (in severe cases)	1. Call 9-1-1. You do not need to capture or kill the snake. 2. When possible, carry the person. If alone and capable, walk slowly. 3. **DO NOT** apply a pressure bandage for a pit viper snakebite; this action has not been proven to be beneficial. According to a number of toxicology associations and the Wilderness Medical Society's Practice Guidelines, the application of pressure bandages for pit viper snakebites is not recommended. 4. *Cautions:* • **DO NOT** cut the person's skin to drain the venom. • **DO NOT** use mouth suction or any suction device. • **DO NOT** apply cold packs or ice packs. • **DO NOT** give alcohol. • **DO NOT** apply electrical shock. • **DO NOT** use a tourniquet.
Coral snakes Identified by: • Small and very colorful, with a series of bright red, yellow, and black bands going all the way around its body Figure 5-6. • Every alternate band is yellow, and the snout is black. • It is the most venomous snake in North America, but rarely bites Figure 5-7.	• Few immediate signs (absence of immediate symptoms is not evidence of a harmless bite) • Several hours may pass before the onset of: • Nausea • Vomiting • Sweating • Tremors • Drowsiness • Slurred speech • Blurred vision • Swallowing difficulty • Breathing difficulty	1. Call 9-1-1. You do not need to capture or kill the snake. 2. Apply a wide elastic bandage using overlapping turns. 3. Start wrapping at the end of the bitten arm or leg and wrap upward, covering its entire length. 4. Use similar tightness as when wrapping a sprained ankle. You should be able to slip a finger under the wrapping. 5. Stabilize the bitten arm or leg as you would for a broken bone and keep it below heart level. 6. **DO NOT** cut skin or use suction.

(continued)

Reptile	What to Look For	What to Do
Nonvenomous snakes If in doubt, assume that the snake is venomous.	• Horseshoe shape of tooth marks on skin • Possible swelling and tenderness	1. Treat the bite the same as you would a shallow wound. (Refer to pages 23-25.) 2. Consult with a physician.
Venomous lizards Includes: • Gila monster (United States and Mexico) • Mexican bearded lizard Identified by: • May firmly hang on during bite and chew venom into skin	• Puncture wounds—teeth may break off • Swelling and pain, often severe and burning • Sweating • Vomiting • Increased heart rate • Shortness of breath	1. Give pain medication. 2. Call 9-1-1. 3. Treat the bite the same you would for a pit viper bite.

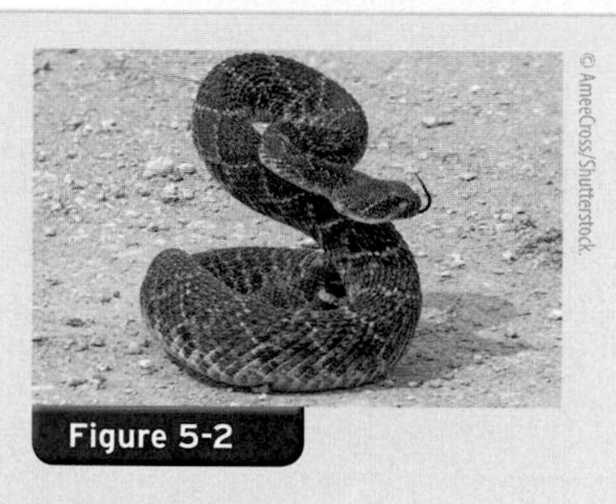

Figure 5-2

Rattlesnake.

© AmeeCross/Shutterstock.

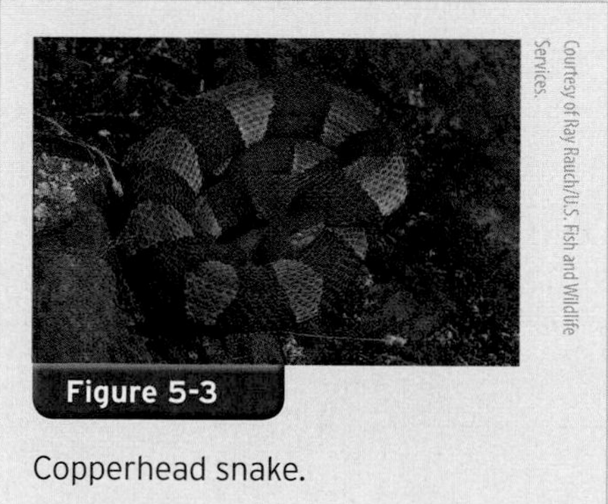

Figure 5-3

Copperhead snake.

Courtesy of Ray Rauch/U.S. Fish and Wildlife Services.

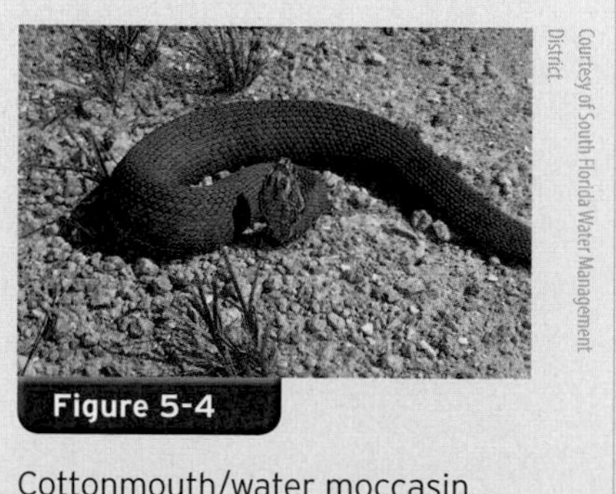

Figure 5-4

Cottonmouth/water moccasin.

Courtesy of South Florida Water Management District.

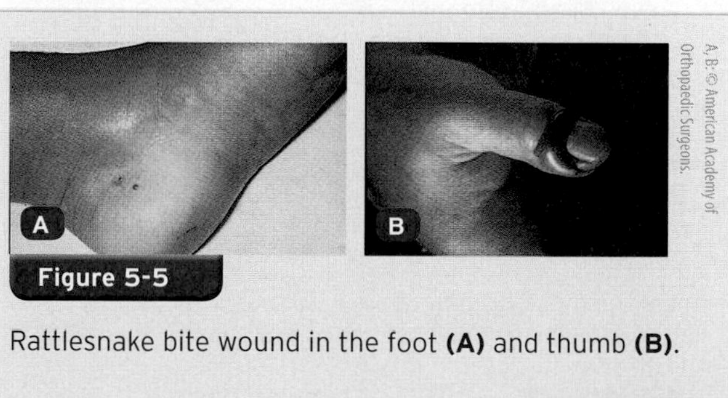

Figure 5-5

Rattlesnake bite wound in the foot **(A)** and thumb **(B)**.

A, B: © American Academy of Orthopaedic Surgeons.

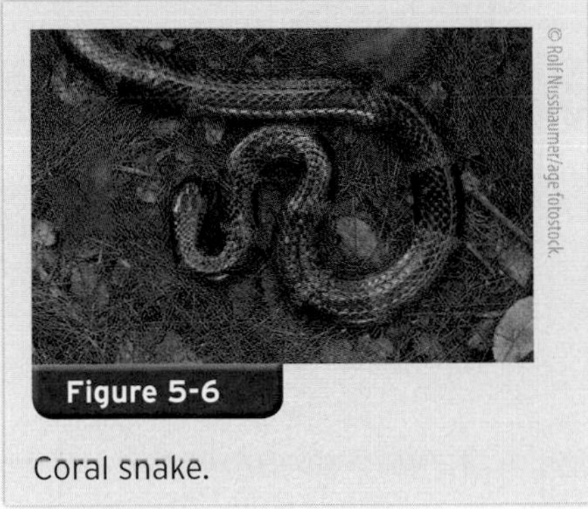

Figure 5-6

Coral snake.

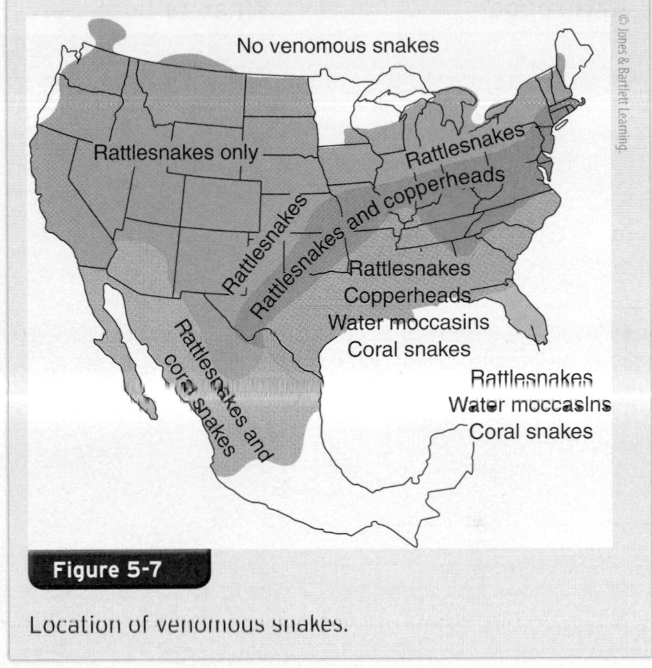

Figure 5-7

Location of venomous snakes.

▶ Arthropod Bites and Stings

Before helping, take the appropriate actions described on pages 5–6.

Arthropods—including scorpions, spiders, centipedes, and ticks—are invertebrates with jointed legs and segmented bodies. Stinging insects cause more deaths than do venomous snakes. People who have had a previous severe reaction should wear a medical identification tag and carry a physician-prescribed epinephrine kit.

Arthropod	What to Look For	What to Do

Stinging insects Figure 5-8
• Honeybee
• Yellow jacket
• Hornet
• Wasp
• Fire ant
	• Usual reactions:
	  • Instant pain, redness, itching Figure 5-9
	• Worrisome reactions:
	  • Hives
	  • Swollen lips/tongue
	  • Tickle in throat
	  • Wheezing
	• Life-threatening reactions:
	  • Blue/gray skin color
	  • Seizures
	  • Unresponsiveness
		1. Look for a stinger; if found, immediately scrape the stinger and venom sac off the skin with a fingernail or plastic card (eg, credit card), or brush it off with your hand. Only bees leave their stinger embedded. **DO NOT** use tweezers. **DO NOT** squeeze the venom sac, which may or may not be attached to the stinger.
		2. Wash the area with soap and water.

(continued)

<table>
<tr><th>Arthropod</th><th>What to Look For</th><th>What to Do</th></tr>
<tr><td></td><td>• Inability to breathe because of swollen vocal cords (cause of about 60% to 80% of anaphylactic deaths)</td><td>3. Apply an ice pack to the area for up to 20 minutes, placing a paper towel or thin damp cloth between the skin and ice pack. Baking soda paste may also help, except for on wasp stings.
4. Give pain medication.
5. Apply hydrocortisone cream (1%) and give an antihistamine (Benadryl) to relieve itching and swelling.
6. For a severe allergic reaction, help the person self-administer epinephrine (see page 58).
7. Monitor breathing, and if it stops, give cardiopulmonary resuscitation (CPR).
8. A sting in the throat or mouth can cause swelling even in a person without an allergy; have the person suck on ice.</td></tr>
<tr><td>Widow spider
Best known as the black widow, but the term black is inaccurate because only three of the five species of widow spiders are black; the others are brown and gray Figure 5-10.
Only adult females bite. They have a shiny, black abdomen with a red or yellow spot that is often in the shape of an hourglass, or white spots or bands on the abdomen.
Most people never see the spider.</td><td>• Sharp pinprick sensation followed by dull, numbing pain
• Two small fang marks seen as tiny red spots
• Severe abdominal pain (bites on an arm can produce severe chest pain, thus mimicking a heart attack)
• Headache, chills, fever, heavy sweating, nausea, and vomiting</td><td>1. Clean with soap and water.
2. Apply an ice pack to the area.
3. Give pain medication.
4. Seek medical care as soon as possible.
5. If facial swelling or anaphylaxis occurs, call 9-1-1 and treat appropriately (see pages 57-58).</td></tr>
</table>

Arthropod	What to Look For	What to Do
Fiddle back spider Also known as brown recluse spider, violin spider, and brown spider **Figure 5-11**	• Mild to severe pain that occurs within 2 to 8 hours • Blister that develops within 48 to 72 hours; becomes red and bursts; takes on a bull's-eye appearance **Figure 5-12** • Nausea, vomiting, headache, and fever	1. Treat the bite the same as you would a black widow spider bite. 2. If the wound becomes infected, apply antibiotic ointment under a sterile dressing. 3. Seek medical care.
Hobo spider Also known as the aggressive house spider	Same as for fiddle back spiders	Treat the bite the same as you would a fiddle back spider bite.
Tarantula spider They bite only when vigorously provoked or roughly handled. They can flick their hairs onto a person's skin **Figure 5-13**.	Varies from mild to severe throbbing pain that lasts up to 1 hour	1. Treat the bite the same as you would a black widow spider bite. 2. For hairs in the skin, remove with sticky tape, wash with soap and water, and apply hydrocortisone cream (1%). 3. Give an antihistamine and pain medication.
Scorpion In the United States, only the bark scorpion found in Arizona is potentially deadly. It is active from May through August.	• Burning pain • Numbness or tingling that occurs later	1. Monitor breathing. 2. Wash with soap and water. 3. Apply an ice pack to the area. 4. Give pain medication. 5. Apply dressing. 6. Seek medical care for severe reactions.
Centipede Do not confuse it with a millipede, which cannot inject venom but can irritate the skin.	• Burning pain • Inflammation • Mild swelling of lymph nodes	1. Clean the wound with soap and water. 2. Apply an ice pack. 3. Give pain medication. 4. If symptoms persist, give an antihistamine (Benadryl) or apply hydrocortisone cream (1%) on the bite site. 5. Most bites will get better even without treatment; however, for severe reactions, seek medical care.

(continued)

<table>
<tr><th>Arthropod</th><th>What to Look For</th><th>What to Do</th></tr>
<tr><td rowspan="2">Tick
Most ticks are harmless, but they can carry diseases (Lyme disease, Rocky Mountain spotted fever, Colorado tick fever, tularemia, etc). The longer the tick stays embedded or the more engorged it is with blood, the greater the chance a disease will be transmitted Figure 5-15.</td><td>• No initial pain; the tick may go unnoticed for days Figure 5-14
• Red area around tick, indicating the tick has punctured the skin and is feeding on the person's blood
• Rash, fever, and chills
• The bite varies from a small bump to extensive swelling and ulcer.</td><td>Ticks are difficult to remove. Partial removal may lead to infection.
To remove the tick:
1. Use tweezers or one of the specialized tick-removal tools to grasp the tick as close to the skin as possible Figure 5-16.
2. Pull upward with steady, even pressure.
3. DO NOT twist or jerk the tick.
4. Lift it to tent the skin surface. Hold in this position until the tick lets go (about 1 minute).
5. Pull tick away from the skin. Try not to pull hard enough to break the tick apart, which leaves parts of the mouth embedded.
6. DO NOT use any of the following ineffective methods to remove the tick:
• Petroleum jelly
• Fingernail polish
• Rubbing alcohol
• Gasoline
• Touching with a blown-out hot match, hot needle, or hot paper clip
7. DO NOT grab a tick at the rear of its body; the tick's internal organs could rupture, resulting in their contents being squeezed into the person.</td></tr>
<tr><td>When the tick is completely removed</td><td>1. Wash your hands and the area with soap and water. Apply rubbing alcohol to further disinfect the area.
2. Apply an ice pack to reduce pain.
3. Apply calamine lotion or hydrocortisone cream to relieve itching.</td></tr>
</table>

Arthropod	What to Look For	What to Do
		4. Place the tick in a plastic bag and bring it to a physician within 72 hours for identification and possible antibiotic treatment in order to prevent serious illness such as Lyme disease. 5. If a rash, fever, or flulike symptoms (headache, body aches, and/or nausea) occur in 3 to 30 days after the tick's removal, seek medical care—with or without the tick.
	Tick's mouth parts broke off and remain in the skin	1. If unable to remove the parts easily, leave them in place and treat with warm soaks and antibiotic ointment. The retained parts will usually expel and the skin will heal. 2. If infection develops, seek medical care.
Chigger mite Bites can number in the hundreds.	• Severe itching that occurs after several hours • Small red welts • Skin infection	1. Wash with soap and water and rinse several times. 2. Apply an ice pack to the area. 3. Apply hydrocortisone cream (1%) or calamine lotion. 4. Give an antihistamine (Benadryl).
Mosquito	• Itching • Mild swelling	1. Wash the affected area with soap and water. 2. Apply an ice pack. 3. Apply calamine lotion or hydrocortisone cream (1%) to decrease itching. 4. For a person with numerous stings or a delayed allergic reaction, an antihistamine (Benadryl) every 6 hours or a physician-prescribed cortisone might be helpful.
Flea	• Itching • Multiple bites—termed "breakfast, lunch, and dinner"	1. Apply an ice pack. 2. Apply hydrocortisone cream (1%). 3. Give an antihistamine (Benadryl).

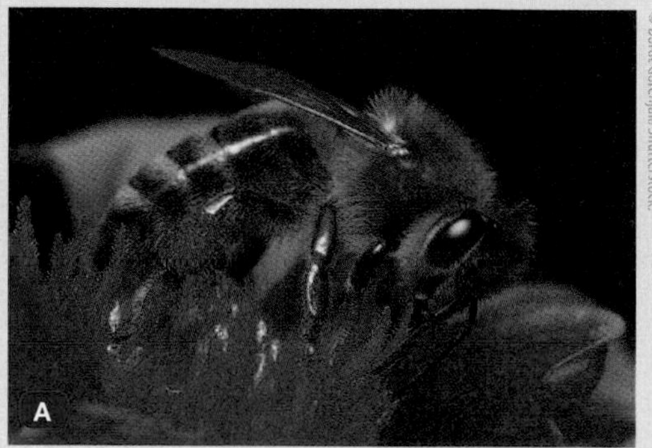

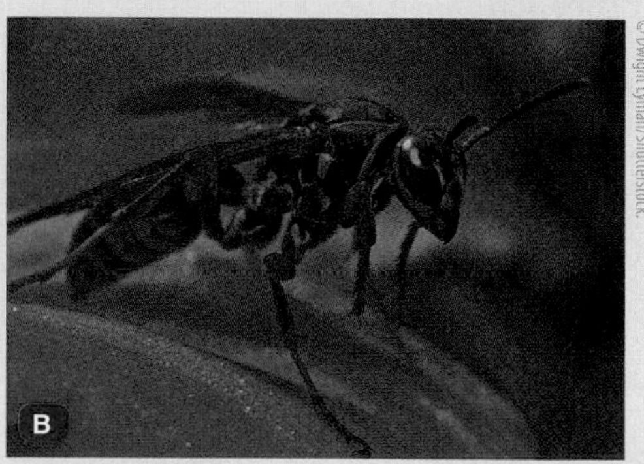

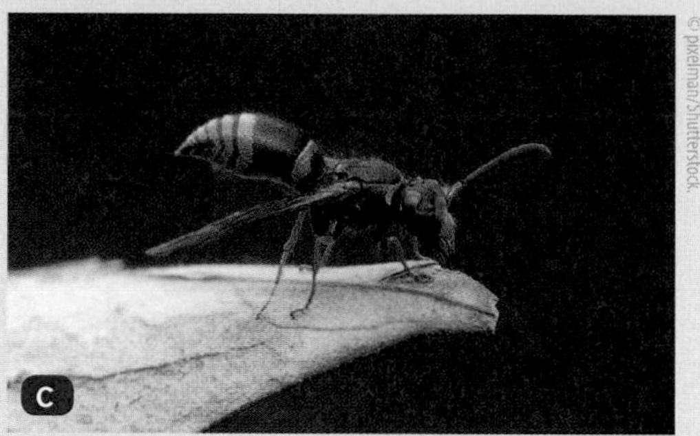

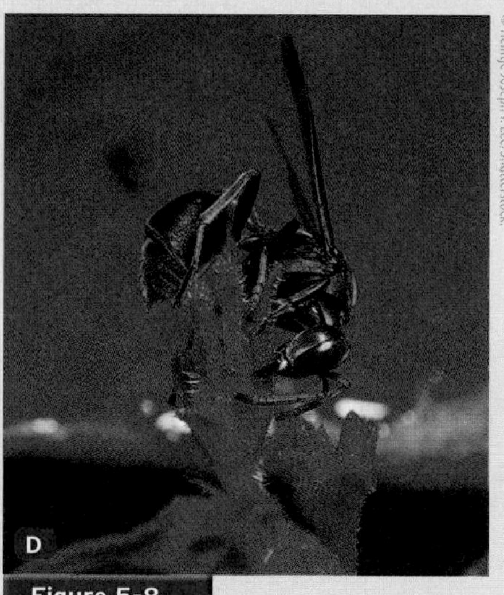

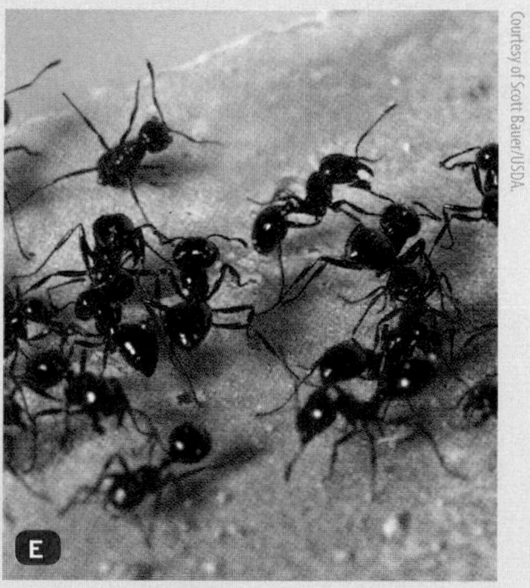

Figure 5-8

Stinging insects. **A.** Honeybee. **B.** Yellow jacket. **C.** Hornet. **D.** Wasp. **E.** Fire ants.

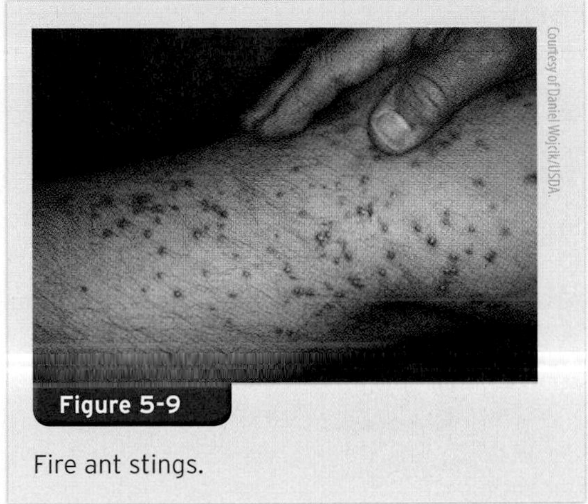

Courtesy of Daniel Wojcik/USDA.

Figure 5-9

Fire ant stings.

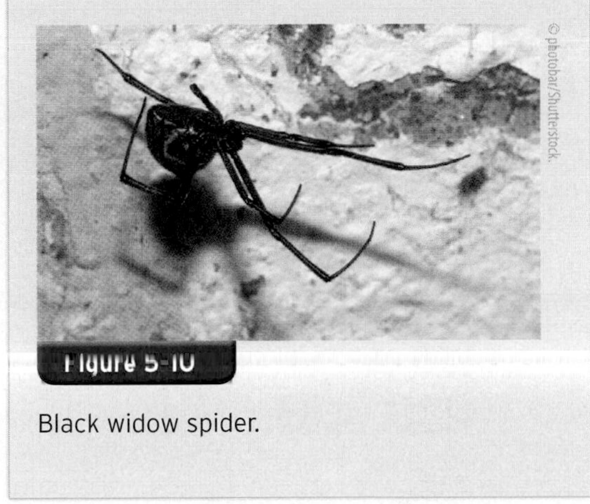

© photobar/Shutterstock.

Figure 5-10

Black widow spider.

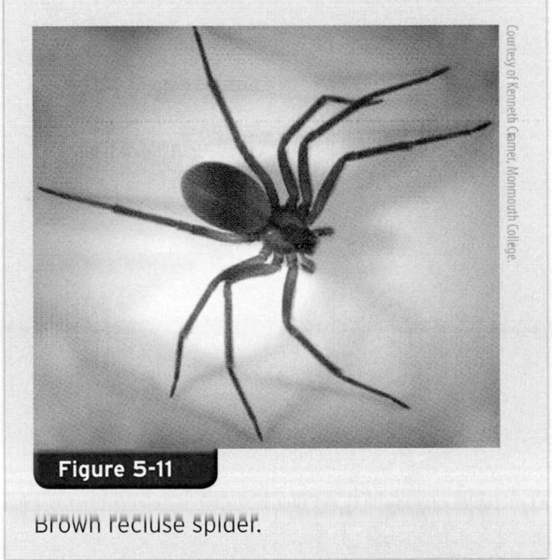

Courtesy of Kenneth Cramer, Monmouth College.

Figure 5-11

Brown recluse spider.

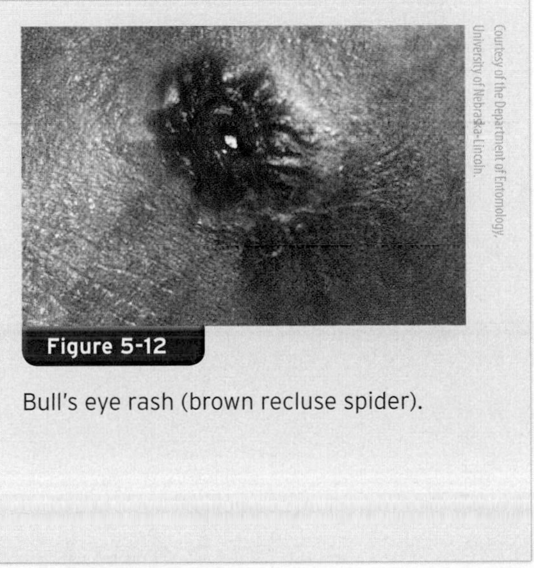

Courtesy of the Department of Entomology, University of Nebraska-Lincoln.

Figure 5-12

Bull's eye rash (brown recluse spider).

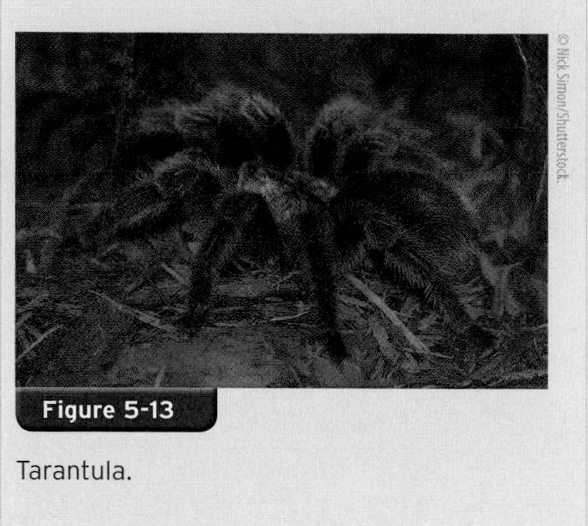

Figure 5-13

Tarantula.

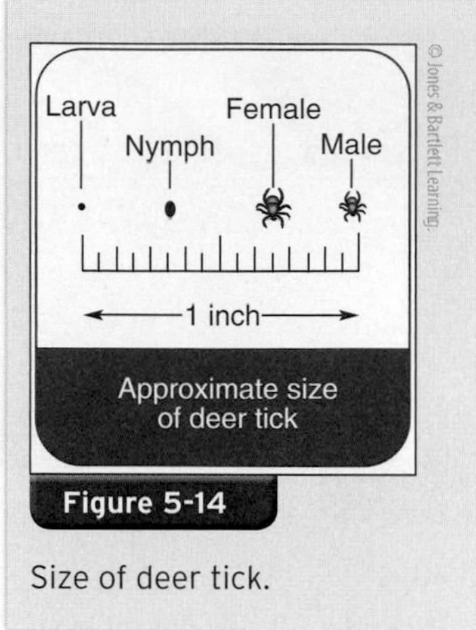

Figure 5-14

Size of deer tick.

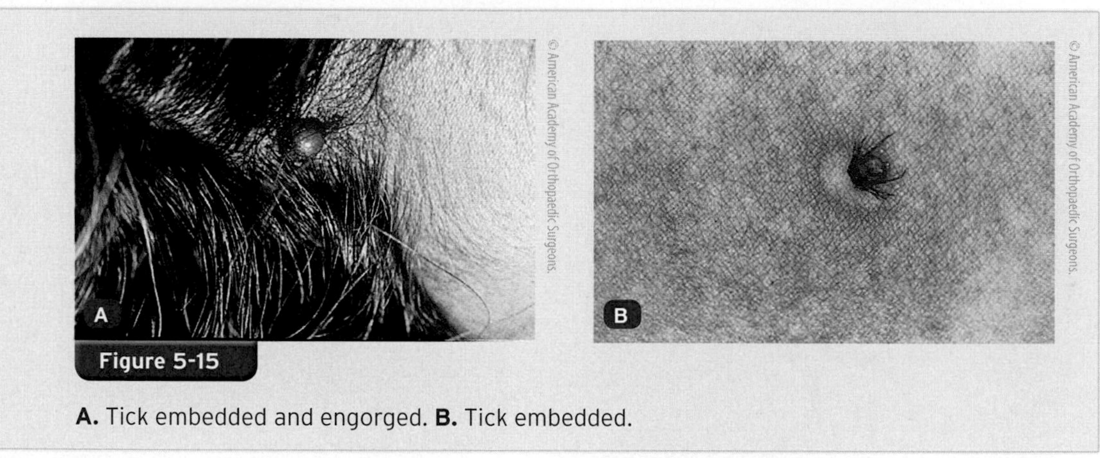

Figure 5-15

A. Tick embedded and engorged. **B.** Tick embedded.

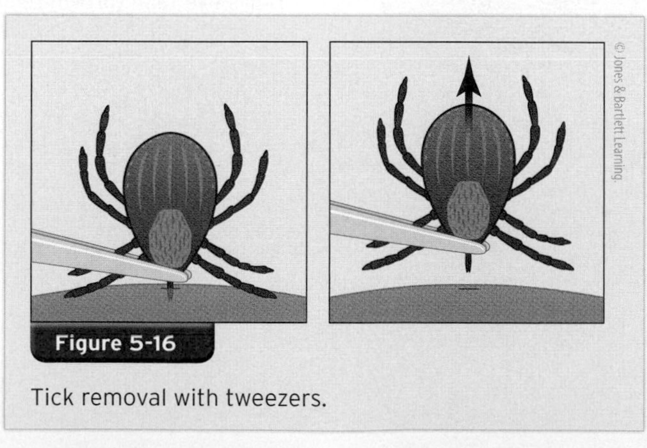

Figure 5-16

Tick removal with tweezers.

▶ Marine Animal Injuries

Before helping, take the appropriate actions described on pages 5–6.

Summon lifeguards or call 9-1-1 if the person is not breathing, if he or she has severe bleeding or signs of a severe allergic reaction such as trouble breathing, or if the face or a large body area has been affected.

A treatment useful for one jellyfish species may worsen the sting from another jellyfish species. This contributes to confusion about what treatment is best. For example, controversy exists about whether vinegar should be used to treat jellyfish stings. According to a review in the *Annals of Emergency Medicine*, 19 reputable medical articles found vinegar increases pain or nematocyst discharge in most jellyfish species in North America and therefore should not be used. Check with local experts, if possible.

Injury Type	Marine Animal	What to Do
Bite, rip, or puncture	• Sharks Figure 5-17 • Barracudas • Eels • Seals	1. Monitor breathing. 2. Control bleeding. 3. Wash wound with soap and water. 4. Flush the area with water under pressure. 5. Treat for shock.
Sting	• Jellyfish Figure 5-18 • Portuguese man-of-wars Figure 5-19 • Sea anemone • Fire coral	**For North American species:** 1. Wash tentacles off with ocean water. **DO NOT** use fresh water. 2. Controversy exists about the use of vinegar for jellyfish stings; what works for one species may make another worse. For only Hawaiian box jellyfish and Portuguese man-of-wars, soak the area in vinegar for 30 seconds. 3. Remove clinging tentacles quickly with tweezers or by scraping with a credit card, razor blade, or clean stick. 4. For all jellyfish stings in North America and Hawaii, soak the area in non-scalding hot water for 20 minutes. Xylocaine (Lidocaine), an OTC medication, can be applied on the affected skin. 5. **DO NOT** use the following remedies: human urine, meat tenderizer, alcohol, and pressure bandages.
Sting	• Sea snake • Octopus • Cone snail	1. Monitor breathing. 2. Control bleeding. 3. Apply pressure bandage on entire arm or leg.

(continued)

Injury Type	Marine Animal	What to Do
Puncture (by spine)	• Stingray Figure 5-20 • Scorpion fish • Stonefish • Starfish • Catfish	1. Soak the area in hot water for 30 to 90 minutes or until pain subsides. **DO NOT** use water that is hot enough to burn. 2. Remove pieces of debris with tweezers. 3. Wash the wound with soap and water. 4. Flush the area with water under pressure. 5. Treat the wound.

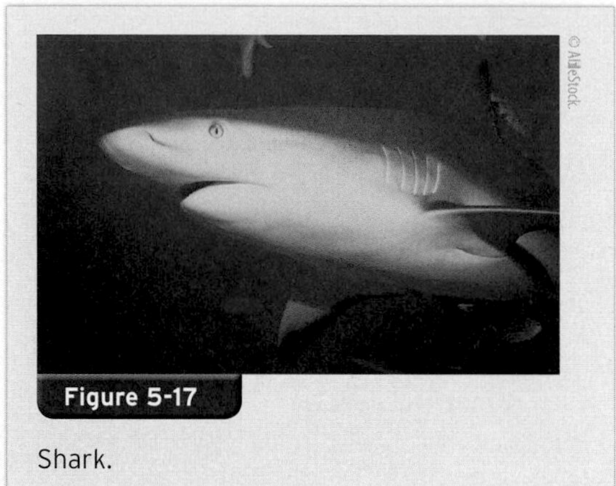

© AbleStock.

Figure 5-17

Shark.

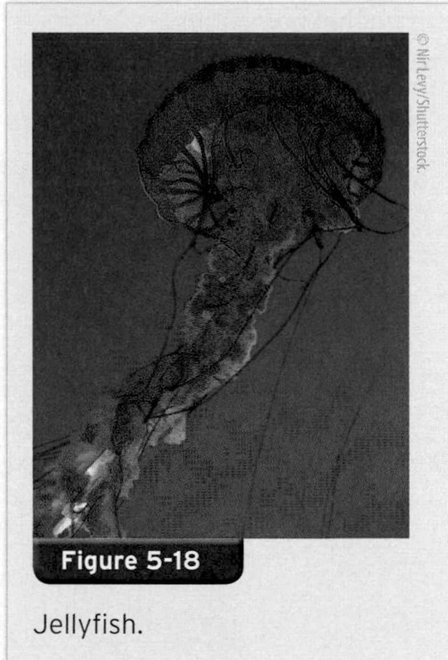

© Nir Levy/Shutterstock.

Figure 5-18

Jellyfish.

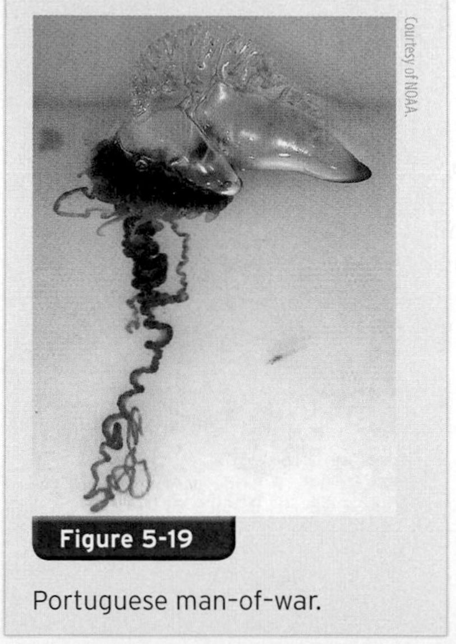

Courtesy of NOAA.

Figure 5-19

Portuguese man-of-war.

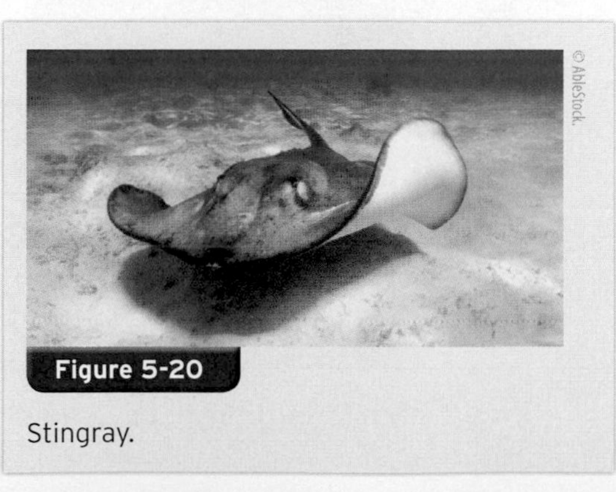

© AbleStock.

Figure 5-20

Stingray.

Temperature (°F)

Relative Humidity (%)	80	82	84	86	88	90	92	94	96	98	100	102	104	106	108	110
40	80	81	83	85	88	91	94	97	101	105	109	114	119	124	130	136
45	80	82	84	87	89	93	96	100	104	109	114	119	124	130	137	
50	81	83	85	88	91	95	99	103	108	113	118	124	131	137		
55	81	84	86	89	93	97	101	106	112	117	124	130	137			
60	82	84	88	91	95	100	105	110	116	123	129	137				
65	82	85	89	93	98	103	108	114	121	128	136					
70	83	86	90	95	100	105	112	119	126	134						
75	84	88	92	97	103	109	116	124	132							
80	84	89	94	100	106	113	121	129								
85	85	90	96	102	110	117	126	135								
90	86	91	98	105	113	122	131									
95	86	93	100	108	117	127										
100	87	95	103	112	121	132										

Likelihood of Heat Disorders with Prolonged Exposure or Strenuous Activity

Caution | Extreme Caution | Danger | Extreme Danger

Courtesy of NOAA.

Figure 5-21

Heat index chart.

▶ Heat-Related Emergencies

Heat illnesses include a range of disorders. Some are common, but only heat stroke is life threatening. Untreated heat stroke results in death. The heat index compiled by the National Weather Service lists the likelihood of heat illnesses at various combinations of temperature and humidity **Figure 5-21**.

Heat Stroke

There are two types of heat stroke: classic and exertional. The common characteristics of classic heat stroke are as follows:

- It is more likely to occur in:
  - Older people
  - People who are chronically ill or sedentary
  - People who take certain prescription medications
  - People who are abusing drugs or alcohol
- It is common during heat waves.
- Affected people do not sweat.

The common characteristics of exertional heat stroke are as follows:

- It affects young, healthy people who are not acclimatized to the heat.
- It usually occurs during strenuous activity.
- Sweating is prevalent in about 50% of affected people.

Heat stroke is life threatening and must be treated rapidly!

What to Look For	What to Do
• Extremely hot skin when touched—usually dry, but may be wet from sweating related to strenuous work or exercise • Altered mental status ranging from slight confusion, agitation, and disorientation to unresponsiveness	1. Move the person from the hot environment to a cool, shaded area. 2. Remove clothing, down to the person's underwear. 3. Cool the person quickly by any means possible. In some remote locations, this might be difficult. **DO NOT** delay cooling the person if any of the following methods (given in the order of effectiveness) are possible: • Whole-body cold water immersion: Place the person in cold water, up to the neck. **DO NOT** leave the person alone. • Evaporative cooling: Spray or douse cold water on the skin and vigorously fan. • Place ice packs against the person's armpits, groin, and sides of the neck. 4. **DO NOT** give aspirin or acetaminophen, as they are ineffective in reducing the body temperature for heat stroke. 5. Stop cooling when mental status improves. 6. Monitor the person frequently, as high temperatures can rise again after cooling. 7. Call 9-1-1 as soon as possible.

Heat Exhaustion

Heat exhaustion differs from heat stroke because the person has no altered mental status and his or her skin is clammy, not hot. However, like heat stroke, you should still cool the person, just not as aggressively as for heat stroke. Recovery may take up to 24 hours.

What to Look For	What to Do
• Sweating • Thirst • Fatigue • Flulike symptoms (headache, body aches, and nausea) • Shortness of breath • Rapid heart rate	1. Move the person to a cool place. 2. Remove excess clothing. 3. Spray or douse cold water on the person's skin and vigorously fan. 4. If the person is able to swallow, give a commercial sports drink, fruit juice, or lightly salted water; if none of these options are available, give cold water. **DO NOT** give salt tablets. 5. Call 9-1-1 if improvement does not occur within 30 minutes. Heat exhaustion can turn into heat stroke.

Hyponatremia (Water Intoxication)

Hyponatremia, also known as water intoxication, may occur when a person drinks too much water, flushing sodium out of the body. Sodium loss is seldom a problem unless the person sweats profusely for long periods of time and drinks large quantities of water.

What to Look For	What to Do
• The person drank too much water (>1 quart [about 1 L] per hour) • Frequent urination; urine is clear • Profuse sweating for long periods • Dizziness, weakness, nausea, vomiting, headache • Altered mental status • Severe sodium loss may result in seizures or unresponsiveness and can be fatal.	1. Move the person to a cool location. 2. **DO NOT** give more fluids. 3. Give salty foods. **DO NOT** give salt tablets because they can irritate the stomach and cause nausea and vomiting. 4. For a person with altered mental status, call 9-1-1 as soon as possible.

Heat Cramps

What to Look For	What to Do
Painful muscle spasms affecting the muscle in the back of the leg or abdomen that happen suddenly during or after physical exertion	Relief may take several hours. 1. Have the person rest in a cool area. 2. Give lightly salted cool water (dissolve 1/4 teaspoon [1.25 mL] salt in 1 quart [about 1 L] of water) or a commercial sports drink. **DO NOT** give salt tablets. 3. Stretch any cramped muscle.

Heat Syncope

What to Look For	What to Do
Dizziness or fainting that occurs immediately after strenuous physical activity in a hot environment	1. If the person is unresponsive, check his or her breathing. A person with heat syncope will usually recover quickly. 2. If the person fell, check for injuries. 3. Have the person rest and lie down in a cool area. 4. Wet the skin with a cool, damp cloth or a spray bottle. 5. If the person is not nauseated and is fully alert and able to swallow, give lightly salted cool water (dissolve 1/4 teaspoon [1.25 mL] salt in 1 quart [about 1 L] of water) or a commercial sports drink. **DO NOT** give salt tablets.

Heat Edema

What to Look For	What to Do
Swollen ankles and feet that occur during the first few days in a hot environment	1. Have the person wear support stockings. 2. Elevate the person's legs.

Heat Rash (Prickly Heat)

What to Look For	What to Do
Itchy rash on skin that is wet from sweating; this condition is seen in humid regions after prolonged sweating.	1. Dry and cool the person's skin. 2. Limit heat exposure.

▶ Cold-Related Emergencies

Hypothermia

Before helping, take the appropriate actions described on pages 5–6.

Hypothermia does not require subfreezing temperatures **Figure 5-22**. It occurs when the body's temperature (98.6°F [37°C]) drops more than 2 degrees. Severe hypothermia is life threatening. Check for possible frostbite.

Treat a person with hypothermia as follows:

1. Stop the heat loss:
   - Get the person out of the cold.
   - Handle the person gently.
   - Replace wet clothing with dry clothing.
   - Add insulation (eg, blankets, towels, pillows, sleeping bags) beneath and around the person. Cover the person's head.
   - Cover the person with a vapor barrier (eg, tarp, plastic, trash bags) to prevent heat loss. **DO NOT** cover the mouth and/or nose. If unable to remove wet clothing, place a vapor barrier between clothing and insulation. For a person who is dry, the vapor barrier can be placed outside the insulation.
2. Keep the person in a flat (horizontal) position.

Additional cautions for hypothermic care are as follows:

- **DO NOT** give a person with altered mental status and decreased responsiveness any warm drinks, as this may cause choking and inhalation of the liquid. If the person is responsive enough to swallow, give him or her warm, sugary drinks; these will help by providing more calories to burn.
- **DO NOT** rub the extremities.
- **DO NOT** place the person in a shower or bath.

Wind Chill Chart

Effective 11/01/01

Wind (mph) \ Temperature (°F)	40	35	30	25	20	15	10	5	0	-5	-10	-15	-20	-25	-30	-35	-40	-45
5	36	31	25	19	13	7	1	-5	-11	-16	-22	-28	-34	-40	-46	-52	-57	-63
10	34	27	21	15	9	3	-4	-10	-16	-22	-28	-35	-41	-47	-53	-59	-66	-72
15	32	25	19	13	6	0	-7	-13	-19	-26	-32	-39	-45	-51	-58	-64	-71	-77
20	30	24	17	11	4	-2	-9	-15	-22	-29	-35	-42	-48	-55	-61	-68	-74	-81
25	29	23	16	9	3	-4	-11	-17	-24	-31	-37	-44	-51	-58	-64	-71	-78	-84
30	28	22	15	8	1	-5	-12	-19	-26	-33	-39	-46	-53	-60	-67	-73	-80	-87
35	28	21	14	7	0	-7	-14	-21	-27	-34	-41	-48	-55	-62	-69	-76	-82	-89
40	27	20	13	6	-1	-8	-15	-22	-29	-36	-43	-50	-57	-64	-71	-78	-84	-91
45	26	19	12	5	-2	-9	-16	-23	-30	-37	-44	-51	-58	-65	-72	-79	-86	-93
50	26	19	12	4	-3	-10	-17	-24	-31	-38	-45	-52	-60	-67	-74	-81	-88	-95
55	25	18	11	4	-3	-11	-18	-25	-32	-39	-46	-54	-61	-68	-75	-82	-89	-97
60	25	17	10	3	-4	-11	-19	-26	-33	-40	-48	-55	-62	-69	-76	-84	-91	-98

Calm

Frostbite Times: 30 minutes, 10 minutes, 5 minutes

Wind Chill (°F) = $35.74+0.6215T - 35.75 (V^{0.16}) + 0.4275T (V^{0.16})$

Where, T=Air Temperature (°F) V=Wind Speed (mph)

Courtesy of the National Weather Service/NOAA.

Figure 5-22

Wind chill chart.

Mild Hypothermia

What to Look For

- Vigorous, uncontrollable shivering. Shivering is desirable because it generates heat that will rewarm the person with mild hypothermia.
- The "umbles"—grumbles, mumbles, fumbles, stumbles, tumbles
- Cool or cold skin on abdomen, chest, or back

What to Do

1. Follow the previously stated steps for treating a person with hypothermia.
2. Apply heat to the chest, armpits, and back (in that order). Use large electric pads, electric blankets, or warm water bottles. Place insulation between the skin and heat source to prevent burning the skin.
3. Give warm, sugary drinks, which can provide energy (calories) and a psychologic boost. These drinks will not provide enough warmth to rewarm the person.
4. **DO NOT** give the person alcohol to drink; it dilates blood vessels, allowing more heat loss.
5. **DO NOT** allow the person to use tobacco.
6. If the person is adequately rewarmed and has a normal mental status, you will usually not need to evacuate him or her to medical care.

Severe Hypothermia

What to Look For	What to Do
• Rigid and stiff muscles • No shivering • Skin feels ice cold and appears blue • Altered mental status • Slow heart rate • Slow breathing rate • The person may appear to be dead	1. Follow the previously stated steps for treating a person with hypothermia. 2. Cut off the person's wet clothing. 3. Monitor the person's breathing, and give CPR if necessary. **DO NOT** start CPR if: • The person has been submerged in cold water for more than 1 hour. • The person has obvious fatal injuries. • The person is frozen (eg, ice in airway). • The person has a chest that is stiff or that cannot be compressed. • Rescuers are exhausted or in danger. 4. Call 9-1-1. 5. Check the person's heart rate for 45 seconds before starting CPR. 6. Provide rewarming if possible by applying heat to the person's chest, armpits, and back (in that order). Use large electric pads or blankets, large chemical heat pads, or warm water bottles. Place insulation between the skin and heat source to prevent burning the skin.

Frostbite

Before helping, take the appropriate actions described on pages 5–6.

Frostbite happens only in below-freezing temperatures and mainly affects the feet, hands, ears, and nose **Figure 5-23**. All frostbite injuries require the same first aid treatment. If frostbite occurs, move the person to a warm place. **DO NOT** let the person walk on frostbitten feet. Remove clothing and jewelry (ie, rings) from the frostbitten body part.

The severity and extent of frostbite are difficult to judge until hours after thawing. The most severe consequences of frostbite occur when tissue dies (gangrene); in cases in which this occurs, the affected part might have to be amputated. The longer the tissue stays frozen, the worse the injury. Check for hypothermia in any person with frostbite. Treat hypothermia and other life-threatening injuries before treating frostbite. Seek medical care as soon as possible.

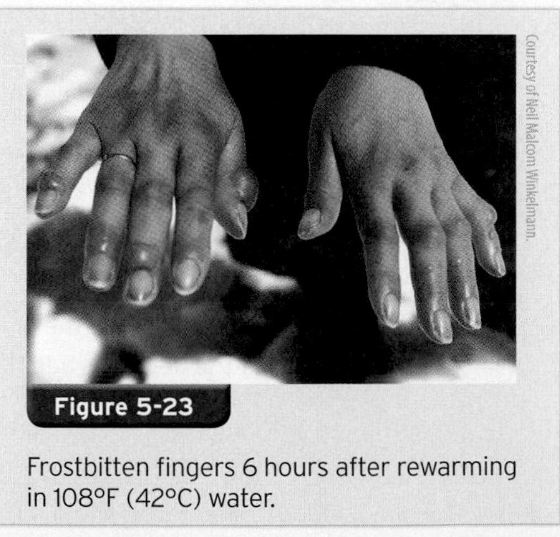

Courtesy of Neil Malcom Winkelmann.

Figure 5-23

Frostbitten fingers 6 hours after rewarming in 108°F (42°C) water.

What to Look For

Before thawing, frostbite can be classified as superficial or deep:

- **Superficial frostbite**
  - White, waxy, or gray-yellow skin
  - The affected part feels very cold and numb. There might be tingling, stinging, or an aching sensation.
  - The skin surface feels stiff or crusty and the underlying tissue feels soft when depressed gently and firmly.
- **Deep frostbite**
  - The affected part feels cold, hard, and solid and cannot be depressed; it feels like a piece of wood or frozen meat.
  - Skin in the affected body part is pale and waxy.
  - A painfully cold part suddenly stops hurting.

What to Do

1. Get the person out of the cold and to a warm place. If possible, do not let the person use a frozen extremity until medical care is reached.
2. Remove any wet clothing and constricting items, such as rings, that could impair blood circulation.
3. **DO NOT** attempt to thaw the part if (a) medical care is less than 2 hours away; (b) the affected area has thawed; (c) shelter, warm water, and a container are not available; or (d) a risk of refreezing exists.
4. Use the wet, rapid rewarming method if (a) medical care is more than 2 hours away; (b) there is no possibility of refreezing the affected area, or (c) shelter, warm water, and a container are available. Although rapid rewarming is recommended, you may be unable to avoid slow thawing; you should allow slow thawing if it is the only method available.
5. *Wet, rapid, rewarming method:* Place the frostbitten part in warm (100°F to 104°F [38°C to 40°C]) water. **DO NOT** use other heat sources (eg, fire, space heater, oven). If you do not have a thermometer, you can put your hand into the water for 30 seconds to test that it is warm but not hot enough to burn. Maintain water temperature by adding warm water as needed. Rewarming usually takes 20 to 40 minutes or until the part becomes soft and pliable to touch and takes on a red/purple appearance. Air dry the area; **DO NOT** rub. To help control the severe pain during rewarming, give the person ibuprofen. For ear or facial injuries, it is best to apply warm, moist cloths, changing them frequently.
6. *Cautions:*
   - **DO NOT** rub or massage the affected area.
   - **DO NOT** apply ice, snow, or cold water to the affected area.
   - **DO NOT** rewarm the affected area with a stove or vehicle's tailpipe exhaust, or over a fire.
   - **DO NOT** break blisters.
   - **DO NOT** allow the person to smoke or drink alcohol.
   - **DO NOT** rewarm if a possibility of refreezing exists.
   - **DO NOT** allow the thawed part to refreeze, as this will result in greater damage (ie, gangrene).

(*continued*)

What to Look For	What to Do

After thawing, frostbite can be categorized by degrees, similar to the classification of burns:
• **First-degree frostbite**
  • The affected part is warm, swollen, and tender.
• **Second-degree frostbite**
  • Blisters form minutes to hours after thawing and enlarge over several days **Figure 5-24**.
• **Third-degree frostbite**
  • Blisters are small and contain red-blue or purple fluid. The surrounding skin may be red or blue and might not blanch when pressure is applied.
	After thawing:
	1. If the feet are affected, do not allow the person to walk. The feet will be impossible to use after they are rewarmed unless only the toes are affected.
	2. Protect the affected area from contact with clothing and bedding.
	3. Place bulky, dry, clean gauze on the affected part and between the toes and the fingers to absorb moisture and keep them from sticking together.
	4. Slightly elevate the affected part above heart level to reduce pain and swelling.
	5. Apply aloe vera gel to promote skin healing.
	6. Give ibuprofen to limit pain and inflammation.
	7. Give fluids if the person is alert and can swallow.
	8. Seek medical care as soon as possible.

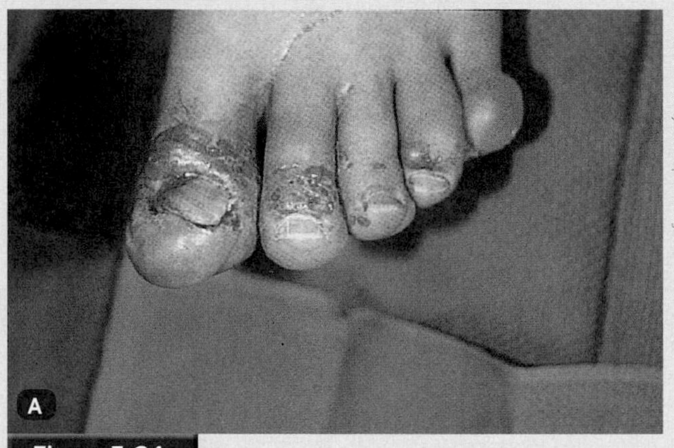

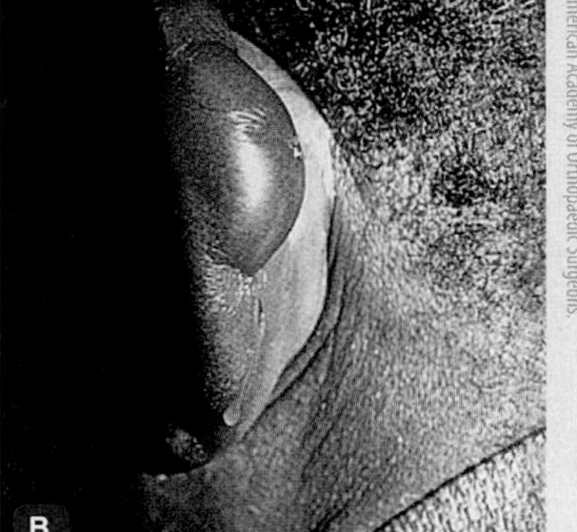

Figure 5-24

Second-degree frostbite of the toe **(A)** and ear **(B)**.

Frostnip

Frostnip is caused when water on the skin surface freezes. It may be difficult to tell the difference between frostnip and frostbite. Frostnip should be taken seriously, as it may be the first sign of impending frostbite.

What to Look For	What to Do
• Yellow to gray skin color • Frost (ice crystals) on the skin • Initial tingling or numbness that may become painful	1. Get the person out of the cold and to a warm place. 2. Gently warm the affected area by placing it against a warm body part (eg, have the person put bare hands under the armpits) or by applying a warm chemical heat pack covered by a cloth. For the nose, breathe with cupped hands over the nose. 3. **DO NOT** rub the area.

▶ Poisoning

Before helping, take the appropriate actions described on pages 5–6.

Swallowed Poisoning

Fortunately, most poisons have little toxic effect or are ingested in such small amounts that severe poisoning rarely occurs. Still, the potential for severe or fatal poisoning is always present.

What to Look For	What to Do
• Abdominal pain and cramping • Nausea or vomiting • Diarrhea • Burns, odor, or stains around and in the mouth • Drowsiness or unconsciousness • Seizure • Poison container nearby	1. Try to determine: • Person's age and weight • Person's condition • What poison was swallowed • When the poison was taken • How much was taken 2. Call the National Poison Control Center hotline at 1-800-222-1222 even if signs of poisoning are not present. 3. Follow their directions. 4. Place the person on his or her left side to delay the poison from moving into the intestines and to prevent inhalation of vomit, if vomiting occurs. 5. Monitor breathing, and if it stops, give CPR. 6. *Cautions:* • **DO NOT** give anything to eat or drink unless advised to do so by the poison control center.

(continued)

What to Look For	What to Do
	• **DO NOT** try to cause vomiting by giving syrup of ipecac or by gagging or tickling the back of the person's throat. • **DO NOT** give activated charcoal unless advised to do so by the poison control center. • **DO NOT** follow the first aid procedures on a container's label. • **DO NOT** give water or milk to dilute poisons other than caustic or corrosive substances (acids and alkalis) unless told to do so by staff at a poison control center. Fluids can dissolve a dry poison, such as tablets or capsules, more rapidly and fill up the stomach, forcing the stomach contents (the poison) into the small intestine, where it will be absorbed faster. Vomiting and aspiration could occur.

Inhaled Poisoning

All affected people require medical care even if they appear to have recovered. If the scene is not dangerous, immediately move the person into fresh air. **DO NOT** enter the scene unless properly equipped and trained.

What to Look For	What to Do

• Headache
• Ringing in the ears (tinnitus)
• Chest pain (angina)
• Muscle weakness
• Nausea and vomiting
• Dizziness and visual changes (blurred or double vision)
• Unresponsiveness
• Respiratory and cardiac arrest
• Indications of possible carbon monoxide poisoning:
  • Symptoms that come and go
  • Symptoms that worsen or improve in certain places or at certain times of the day
  • Similar symptoms in people around the person who is ill
  • Pets that seem ill
	1. Call 9-1-1 as soon as possible.
	2. Try to determine:
	  • What substance was inhaled
	  • When the exposure occurred
	  • How long the substance was inhaled
	  • The person's condition
	3. Place the person in a sitting or reclining position, or in whatever position best facilitates breathing and is comfortable. Support the back for easier breathing.
	4. Monitor breathing, and if it stops, give CPR.

▶ Poison Ivy, Poison Oak, and Poison Sumac Reactions

Before helping, take the appropriate actions described on pages 5–6.

Poison ivy can be found in every state, except Hawaii and Alaska Figure 5-25. Poison oak grows in some eastern states and along the West Coast Figure 5-26. Poison sumac is found mainly in swampy areas on the East Coast, especially in the Southeast Figure 5-27.

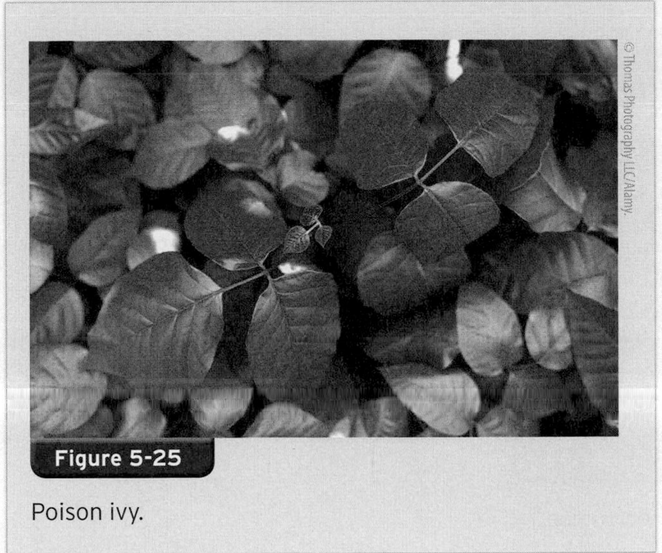

Figure 5-25

Poison ivy.

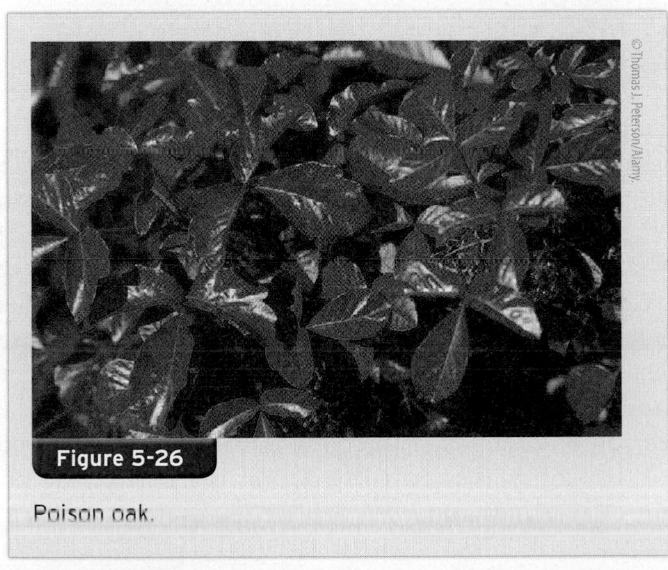

Figure 5-26

Poison oak.

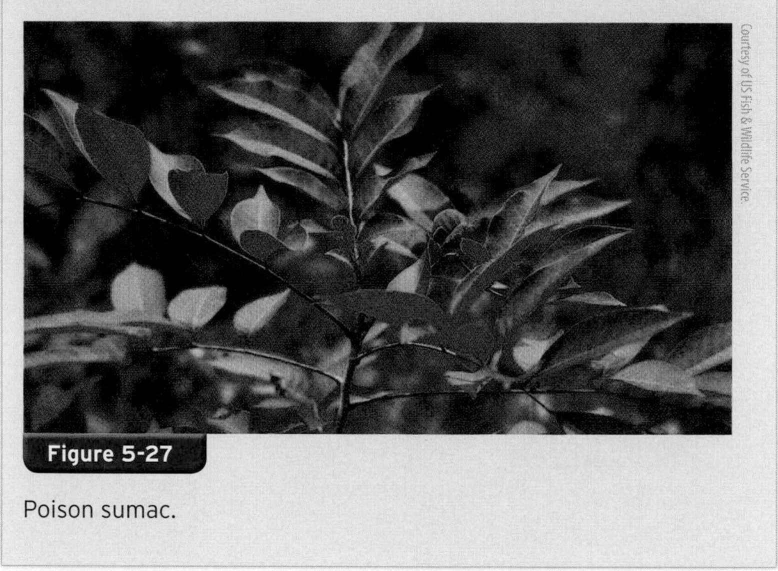

Courtesy of US Fish & Wildlife Service.

Figure 5-27

Poison sumac.

Poison ivy growing in one area may not look anything like poison ivy found halfway across the country, and poison oak of the East Coast is very different from poison oak in the West Coast. However, the dermatitis that these plants cause—and the treatment—is similar Figure 5-28.

The poison in these plants is urushiol, a chemical that is found in the plant's sap. All parts of the plant—leaves, stems, roots, flowers, and berries—contain urushiol oil. About 50% of the people exposed to these plants break out in a rash. An allergic reaction may begin as early as 6 hours after exposure, with a line of small blisters forming where the skin brushed against the plant, followed by redness, swelling, and larger blisters. Usually, the onset of symptoms is 24 to 72 hours after exposure. Following the initial eruption, the rash may appear on other areas of the body for up to 2 weeks. This depends on the amount of urushiol the skin was exposed to and/or the part of the body that absorbed the urushiol.

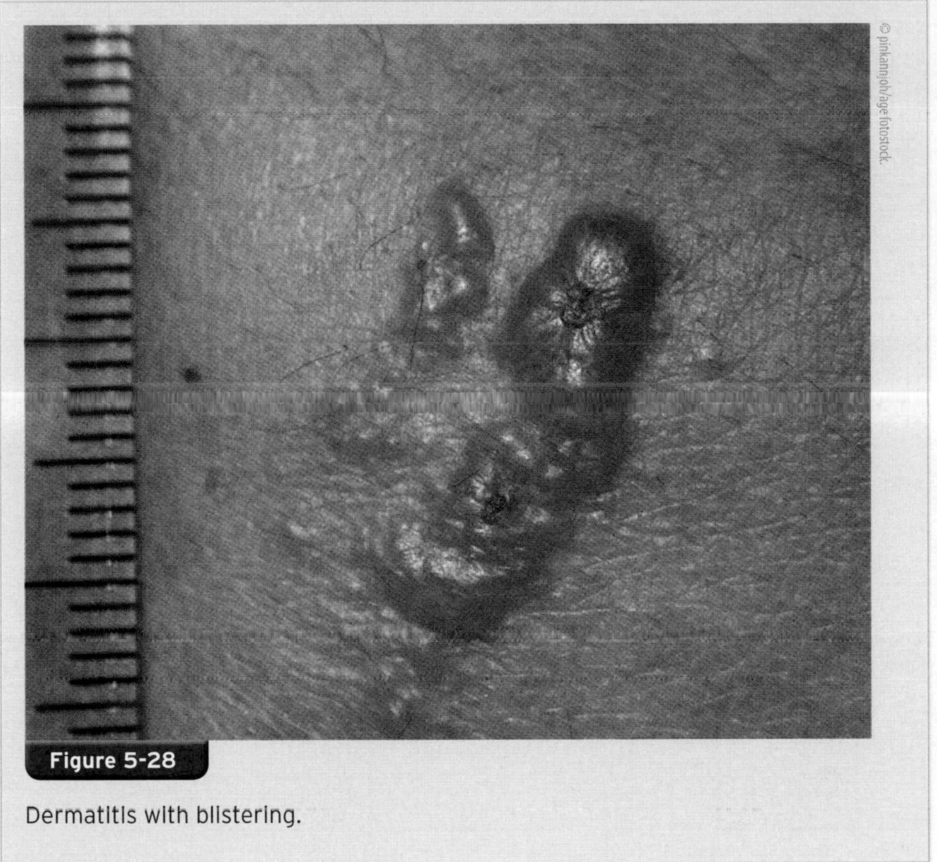

Figure 5-28

Dermatitis with blistering.

Poison ivy, oak, and sumac dermatitis are self-limiting conditions. Without any treatment, a mild case of any of these will often disappear in about 2 weeks. Usually the discomfort is significant, and OTC hydrocortisone cream or ointment (1%) offers little benefit. Although the first aid procedures discussed here will not cure the condition, they will ease the suffering. Seek medical advice for severe cases.

Do not worry about spreading the rash to others; it is not contagious and the blister fluid itself does not contain the irritant. However, the oil or particles of the oil can be carried on the fur of animals and in the smoke of burning plants. Both can affect a person with an allergy.

What to Look For	What to Do
Known contact within 5 minutes for people with sensitive skin and up to 1 hour for people with moderately sensitive skin	If within 5 minutes of an exposure: 1. Gently wipe skin with rubbing alcohol. **DO NOT** rub it in. **DO NOT** use packaged alcohol wipes. 2. Next, or if rubbing alcohol is not available, wash the skin with lots of cold running water. Soap is not necessary, but if used, rinse with lots of cold running water. **DO NOT** scrub skin. 3. **DO NOT** use gasoline.
Mild dermatitis: itching	1. Apply any of the following: • Colloidal oatmeal bath (Aveeno Soothing Bath Treatments) • Baking soda paste (1 teaspoon [5 mL] water mixed with 3 teaspoons [15 mL] baking soda) • Calamine lotion • Aluminum acetate solution (Burow's solution) • Physician-prescribed medication 2. If none of the above are available, the application of OTC hydrocortisone may be beneficial in mild cases.
Moderate dermatitis: itching and swelling	• Treat the same as for mild signs and symptoms. • Apply a physician-prescribed cortisone ointment.
Severe dermatitis: itching, swelling, and blisters	• Treat the same as for mild and moderate symptoms. • Apply a physician-prescribed topical or oral cortisone. • Seek medical care if the person inhales smoke from a burning plant or if the reaction involves the face, eyes, genitals, or large areas of the body.

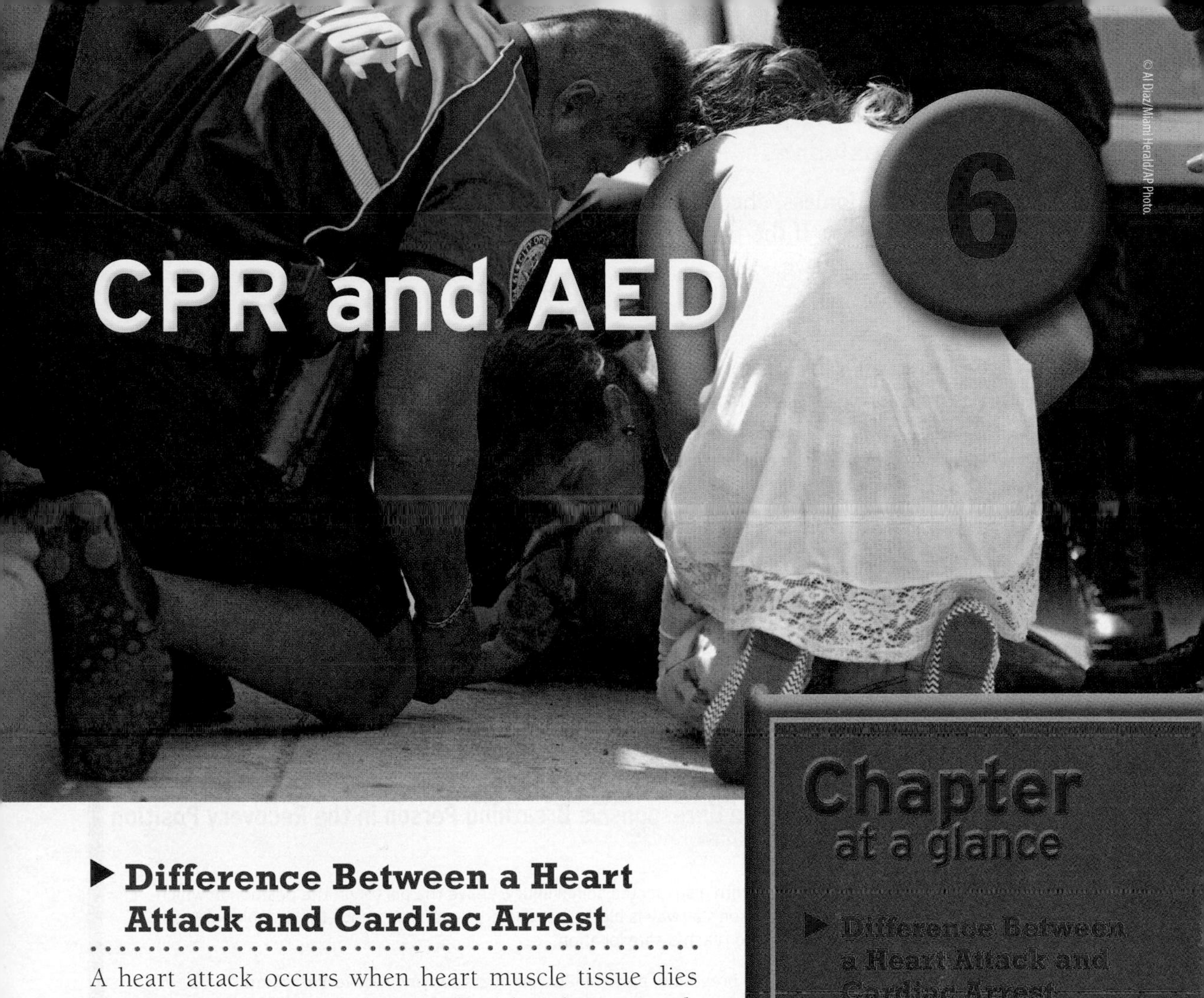

6 CPR and AED

Chapter at a glance

Difference Between a Heart Attack and Cardiac Arrest

A heart attack occurs when heart muscle tissue dies because its blood supply is severely reduced or stopped. This often occurs because of a clot in one or more coronary arteries. First aid for a heart attack is found on page 59.

If damage to the heart muscle is too severe, a person's heart can stop beating—a condition known as cardiac arrest. Sudden cardiac arrest is a leading cause of death.

Performing CPR

When a person's heart stops beating, he or she needs to quickly receive cardiopulmonary resuscitation (CPR), defibrillation, and the help of the emergency medical service (EMS). CPR consists of chest compressions to move blood to the heart and brain and periodic breaths to place oxygen into the lungs. CPR techniques are similar for infants (younger than 1 year), children (1 year to puberty), and adults (puberty and older), with slight variations.

Check for Responsiveness

In a person who is motionless, check for responsiveness by tapping the person's shoulder and asking if he or she is okay. If the person does not respond (ie, does not answer, move, moan, etc), he or she is unresponsive.

Activate EMS

Ask a bystander to call 9-1-1. If you are alone with an adult and a phone is nearby, call 9-1-1 and get an automated external defibrillator (AED). If you are alone with a child or infant, give five sets of 30 chest compressions and two breaths before calling 9-1-1 and getting an AED.

Check Breathing

Place the person faceup on a flat, firm surface. Observe the face and chest movement for breathing. Take 5 seconds but no more than 10 seconds. If the person is not breathing or is only occasionally gasping (may sound like a quick inhalation or like a groan/snore), CPR is needed. If the person is breathing but not responding, CPR is not needed. Place the person in the recovery position to keep the airway clear, and monitor breathing Skill Sheet 6-1.

Skill Sheet

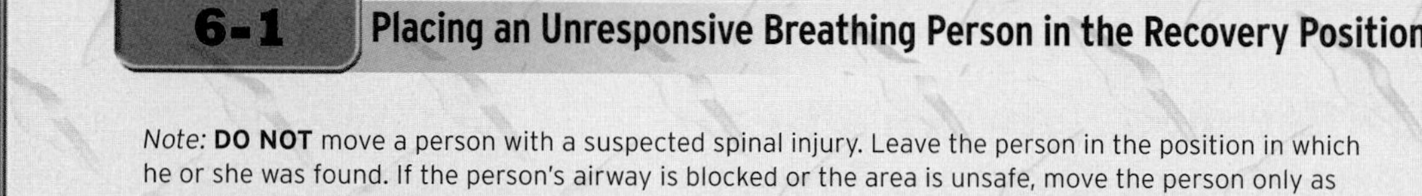

6-1 Placing an Unresponsive Breathing Person in the Recovery Position

Note: **DO NOT** move a person with a suspected spinal injury. Leave the person in the position in which he or she was found. If the person's airway is blocked or the area is unsafe, move the person only as needed to open the airway or to reach a safe location.

If a person is unresponsive and breathing, place him or her in a side-lying recovery position.

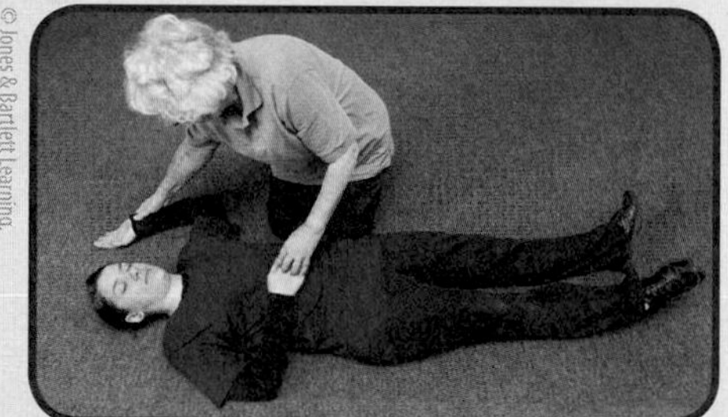

1. Kneel next to the person's side. Straighten both legs. Place the arm nearest you out from the body, with the elbow bent and the palm facing up.

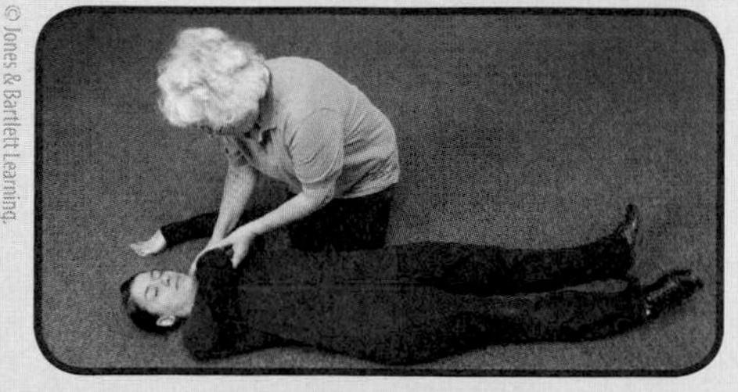

2. Bring the other arm across the person's chest, and place the back of the hand against the cheek nearest you.

Check Out Receipt

Marcy Library
951-826-2078
www.riversideca.gov/library

Thursday, July 20, 2017 2:26:52 PM
27782

Item: 0000143300507
Title: First aid, CPR, and AED. Standard
Call no.: 616.0252 THY 2016
Due: 08/03/2017

Total items: 1

You just saved $15.95 by using your library. You have saved $15.95 this past year and $54.89 since you began using the library!

Thank You!

Skill Sheet Continued

6-1 Placing an Unresponsive Breathing Person in the Recovery Position

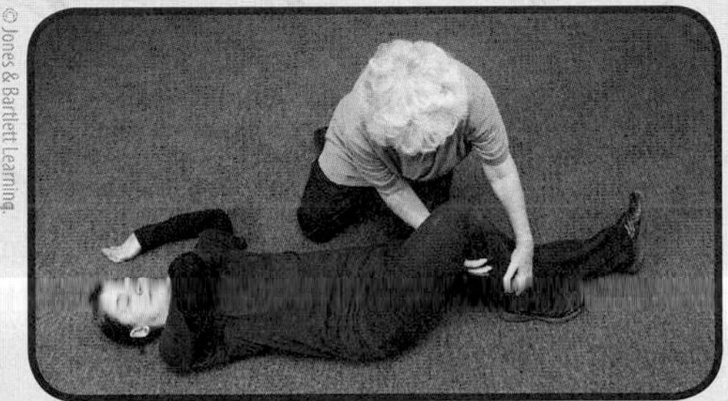

3 Grab and raise the far knee until it is bent, keeping the foot flat on the ground or floor.

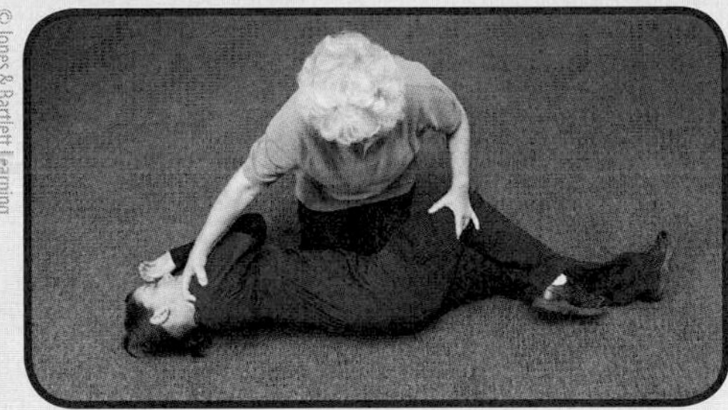

4 Grab the person's bent knee and shoulder, and, with a smooth motion, roll the person toward you, without twisting the body, onto the side.

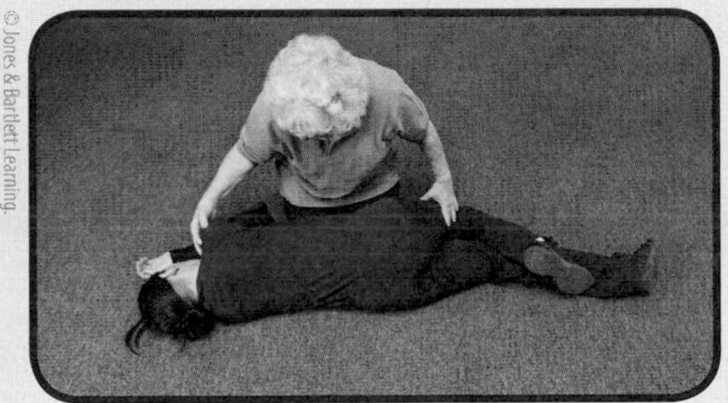

5 Adjust the top leg so that both the knee and hip are bent at right angles. The bent leg and the elbow touching the ground or floor serve as props.

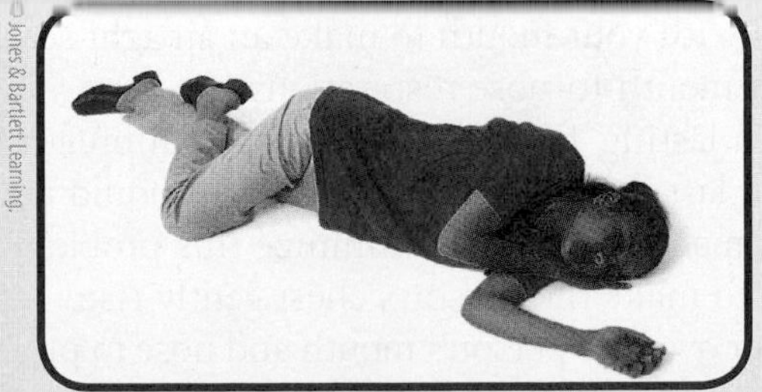

6 Keep the top hand under the person's cheek to cushion it, keep the airway open, and allow fluids to drain.

The advantages of placing an unresponsive, breathing person on his or her side include the following:

- Helps keep the airway open
- Allows fluids (ie, blood, vomit, mucus) to drain out of the nose and mouth and not into the throat
- If you are alone, allows you to leave to call for help

The left-sided recovery position may be preferred for the following reasons:

- Delays vomiting by placing the end of the food pipe (esophagus) above the stomach
- Delays a swallowed poison's effects by retaining the poison in the stomach (A poison can be better dealt with in the stomach than in the small intestines.)
- Relieves pressure on a pregnant woman's vena cava (the body's largest vein)

Give Chest Compressions

Chest compressions are the most important step in CPR and, whenever possible, should be performed on a firm, flat surface. Perform chest compressions with two hands for an adult, one or two hands for a child, and two fingers for an infant. Effective compressions require you to push hard and push fast. Compress the chest of an adult at least 2 inches (5 cm) but no more than 2.4 inches (6 cm); the chest of a child about 2 inches (5 cm) or at least one-third depth of the upper body (chest); and the chest of an infant about 1.5 inches (4 cm) or at least one-third depth of the upper body. For adults and children, compress in the center of the chest and the lower half of the sternum (breast bone). For infants, position two fingers in the center of the chest, both placed below the imaginary nipple line, with the one nearest the head touching the line. After each compression, allow full recoil of the chest. **DO NOT** lean on the chest of an adult or child.

Give compressions at a rate of at least 100 to 120 times per minute for all people receiving CPR. It may be helpful to compress the chest to the beat of the song "Stayin' Alive" by the Bee Gees or to the beats provided by a smartphone app. The app should be previously installed and easily accessible.

Give Breaths

Tilt the person's head back and lift the chin to open the airway. With the airway open, pinch the person's nose shut and make a tight seal over the person's mouth with your mouth. For infants, use the head tilt–chin lift maneuver, but **DO NOT** tilt the head back as far as for an adult or child. Cover the infant's mouth and nose with your mouth to make an airtight seal. If this does not work, try either mouth-to-mouth or mouth-to-nose respirations.

For all people receiving CPR, give one breath lasting 1 second, take a normal breath for yourself, and then give the person another breath lasting 1 second. Each breath should make the person's chest rise. The breaths can cause stomach distension. Minimize this problem by limiting the force of your breath—you only need to make the person's chest gently rise.

A device can be placed in the person's mouth or over the person's mouth and nose to protect against disease transmission. Several different types of barrier devices are available.

Refer to **Skill Sheet 6-2** for the appropriate steps and techniques for adult or child CPR. Refer to **Skill Sheet 6-3** for infant CPR.

Skill Sheet

6-2 Adult and Child CPR

Note: Whenever possible, use a mouth-to-barrier device to prevent disease transmission. Use ***RAB-CAB*** to remember what to do.

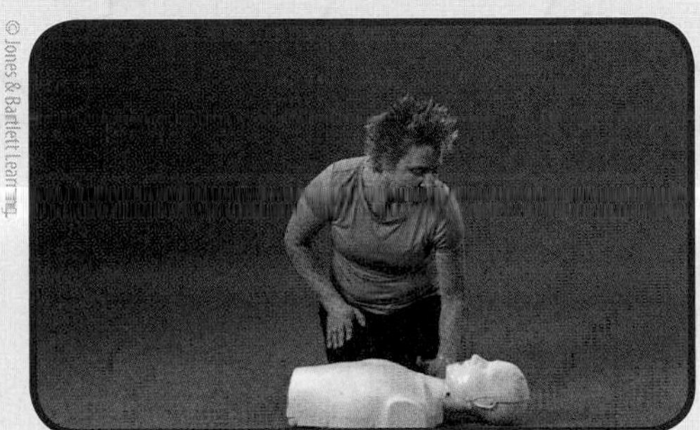

© Jones & Bartlett Learning.

R = Responsive? Tap the person on the shoulder and shout, "Are you okay?"

If the person responds:

- Ask the person about chief complaints.
- Use the SAMPLE (signs and symptoms; allergies; medications; pertinent past medical history; last oral intake; events leading up to the illness or injury) history questions.
- Check the person for DOTS (deformities, open wounds, tenderness, and swelling) if an injury is suspected.

If the person does not respond, continue to Step 2.

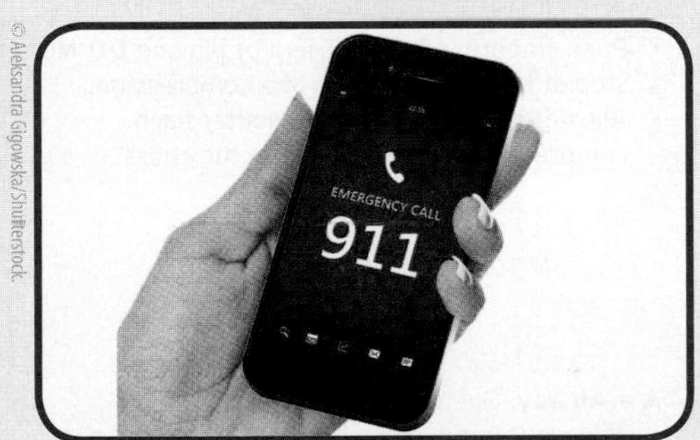

© Aleksandra Gigowska/Shutterstock.

A = Activate EMS. If you are alone:

- Shout for help.
- Activate EMS by calling 9-1-1 or the local emergency number. If a cell phone is used, it should be kept by the person's side, if possible.
- If a cell phone is not available, leave the person to activate EMS and get an AED before starting CPR.

If another person arrives or is nearby, have him or her activate EMS and get an AED.

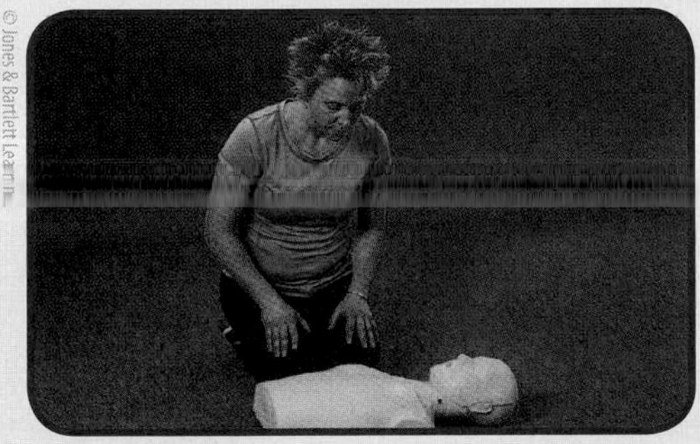

© Jones & Bartlett Learning.

B = Breathing?

- Place the person faceup on a flat, firm surface.
- Observe the person's chest for movement (rise and fall); take 5 sec but no more than 10 sec.
- If the person is not breathing or is only gasping, continue to Step 4.
- If the person is breathing normally, continue to monitor his or her breathing until EMS arrives.

Skill Sheet Continued

6-2 Adult and Child CPR

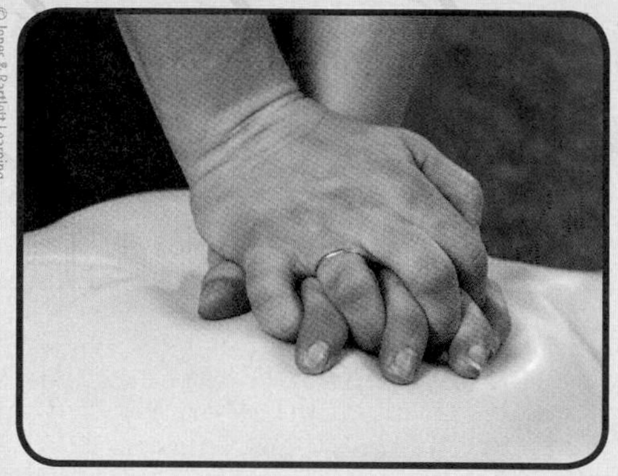

4 **C = Compressions**

- Place the heel of one of your hands on the center of the person's chest and on the lower half of his or her breast bone (sternum).
- Place your other hand on top of the first one with your fingers interlocked. Hold your fingers off the person's chest and point them directly away from you; **DO NOT** cross your hands.
- Keep your arms straight and elbows locked, with your shoulders positioned directly over your hands.
- Push hard: straight down on the sternum, at least 2 in. (5 cm) to 2.4 in. (6 cm) for an adult, or 2 in. (5 cm) or 1/3 depth of the chest for a child.
- Push fast: 100–120 compressions per minute. Consider using the beat of the Bee Gees song "Stayin' Alive."
- Push smoothly: **DO NOT** jerk or jab and **DO NOT** stop at the top or bottom of a compression.
- Allow the chest to fully recoil after each compression (**DO NOT** lean on the chest).

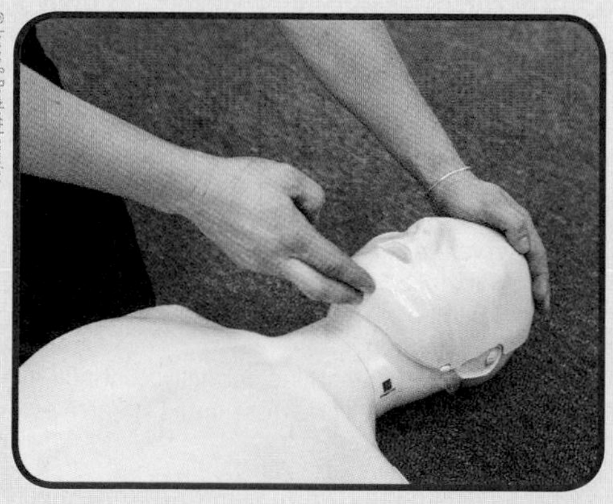

5 **A = Airway**. Open the person's airway.

- Take your hand nearest the person's head and place it on his or her forehead; apply pressure to tilt the head back.
- Place two fingers of your other hand under the bony part of the person's jaw (near the chin) and lift. Avoid pressing on soft tissues under the jaw.
- Tilt the head backward.

Skill Sheet Continued

6-2 Adult and Child CPR

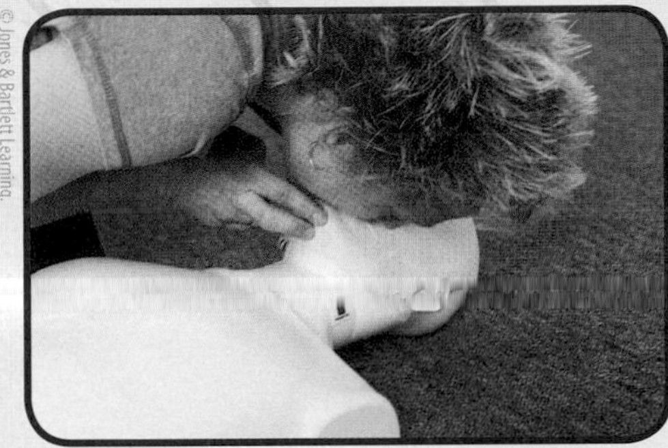

6 **B = Breaths.** Give 2 breaths.

- Pinch the person's nose shut.
- Give 2 breaths, each lasting 1 sec. (Take a normal breath for yourself after each breath.)
- Watch for chest rise to determine if your breaths go in.
- Allow for chest deflation after each breath.
- If you see chest rise after the 2 breaths, give 30 chest compressions.
- If the first breath does not make the chest rise, retilt the person's head and give a second breath. If the second breath does not make the chest rise, begin CPR (30 compressions and 2 breaths). Each time before giving the first of the 2 breaths, open the mouth and look for an object; if seen, remove it.
- If you cannot use the person's mouth (ie, seriously injured mouth, ineffective seal, mouth cannot be opened, person is in water), use the head tilt-chin lift maneuver. Seal your mouth around the person's nose and breathe.

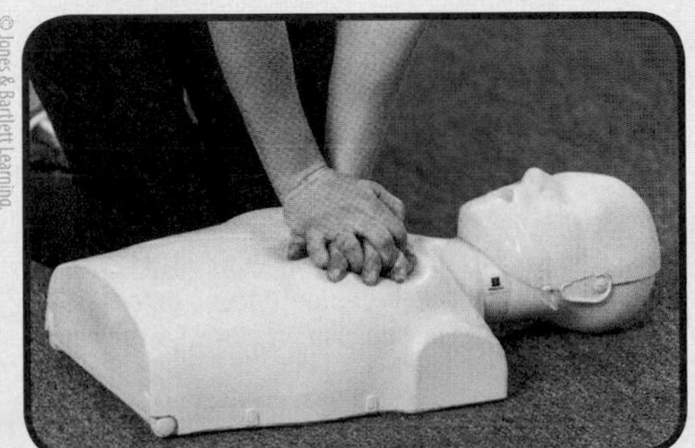

7 Continue sets of 30 chest compressions and 2 breaths until an AED arrives. (If a bystander is present, he or she could help by giving chest compressions while you perform rescue breathing, or vice versa.)

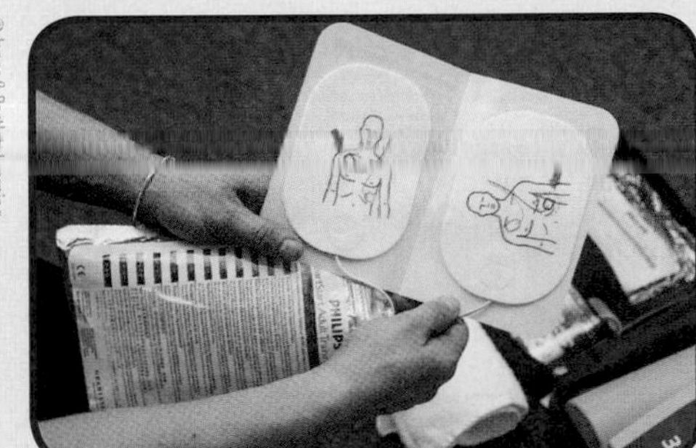

8 When an AED becomes available, use it as soon as possible (see Skill Sheet 6-6).

Skill Sheet

6-3 Infant CPR

Use ***RAB-CAB***.

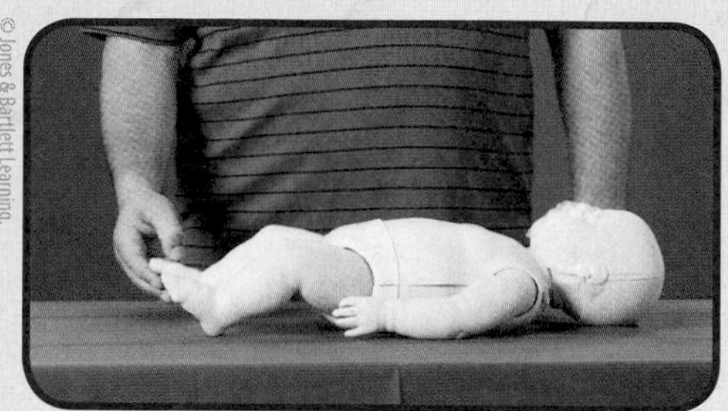

1 **R = Responsive?** Tap the infant's foot and shout his or her name.

- Shout for nearby help.
- Check for no breathing or only gasping.
- Take 5 sec, but no more than 10 sec.

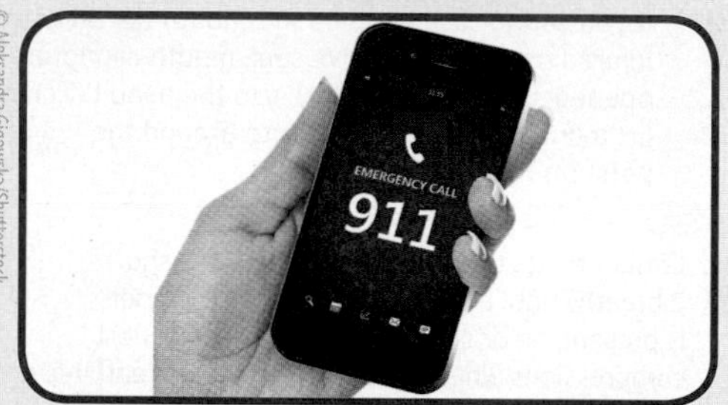

2 **A = Activate** EMS by asking someone to call 9-1-1. If you are alone, **DO NOT** call 9-1-1 until after giving 5 sets of CPR.

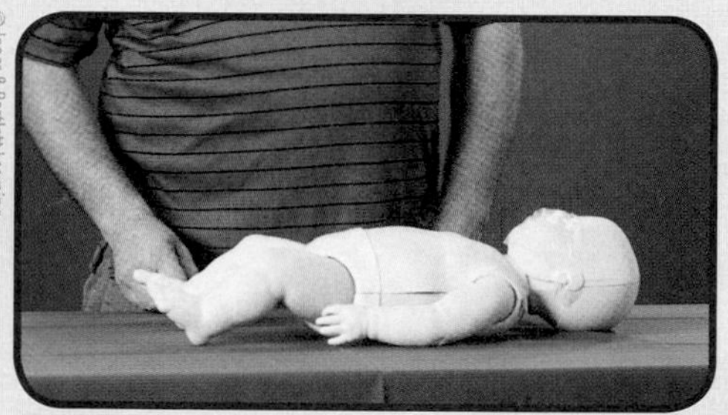

3 **B = Breathing?** Check for no breathing or only gasping by observing the infant's face and chest movement. Position the infant faceup on a flat, firm surface. If possible, use an elevated surface (eg, table, cabinet top).

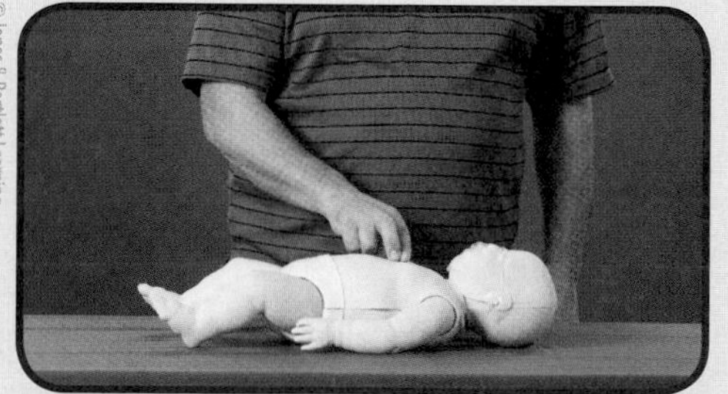

4 **C = Compressions**

- Place the pads of 2 fingers on the infant's breast bone, with 1 touching and both below the nipple line.
- Give 30 chest compressions:
  - Push hard—about 1.5 in. (4 cm) straight down.
  - Push fast—to the beat of the song "Stayin' Alive."
  - At the end of each compression, let the infant's chest come back up to its normal position.

Skill Sheet Continued

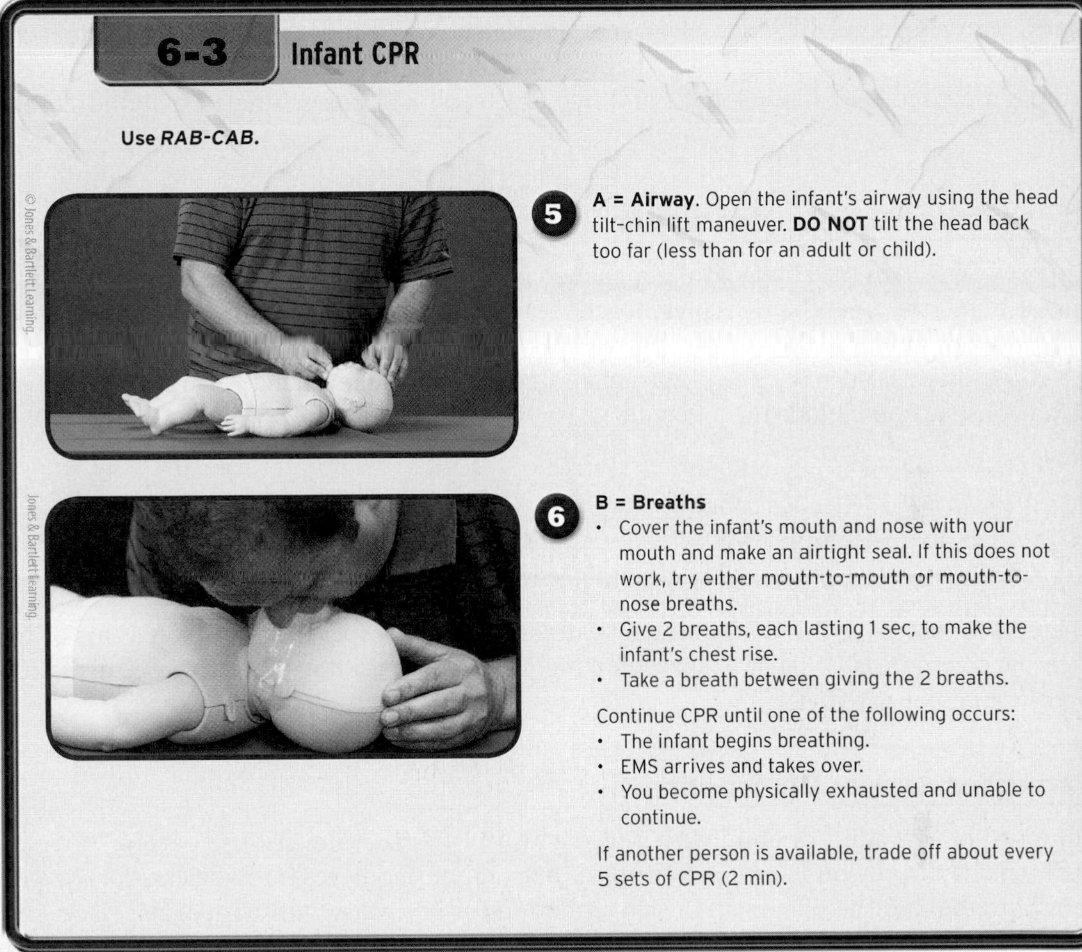

6-3 Infant CPR

Use *RAB-CAB.*

5 **A = Airway.** Open the infant's airway using the head tilt-chin lift maneuver. **DO NOT** tilt the head back too far (less than for an adult or child).

6 **B = Breaths**

- Cover the infant's mouth and nose with your mouth and make an airtight seal. If this does not work, try either mouth-to-mouth or mouth-to-nose breaths.
- Give 2 breaths, each lasting 1 sec, to make the infant's chest rise.
- Take a breath between giving the 2 breaths.

Continue CPR until one of the following occurs:

- The infant begins breathing.
- EMS arrives and takes over.
- You become physically exhausted and unable to continue.

If another person is available, trade off about every 5 sets of CPR (2 min).

▶ Compression-Only CPR

Compression-only CPR intends to increase bystander involvement when CPR is needed for a person in cardiac arrest. Compression-only CPR is easy to teach, remember, and perform compared with conventional CPR.

A bystander who sees a person suddenly collapse and is not breathing but who is unable or unwilling to make mouth-to-mouth contact or is untrained in CPR can:

1. Ask another person to call 9-1-1 or an emergency response number.
2. Push the center of the chest hard and fast (faster than one per second or to the beat of the Bee Gees song "Stayin' Alive").
3. Continue chest compressions without stopping until help arrives or as long as possible. If another person is available, trade off about every 2 minutes.

Airway Obstruction

People can choke on all kinds of objects. Foods such as candy, peanuts, and grapes are major offenders because of their shapes and consistencies. Nonfood choking deaths are often caused by balloons, balls and marbles, toys, and coins inhaled by children and infants.

Recognizing Airway Obstruction

An object lodged in the airway can cause a mild or severe airway obstruction. In a mild airway obstruction, good air exchange is present and the person is able to make forceful coughing efforts in an attempt to relieve the obstruction. The person should be encouraged to cough.

A person with a severe airway obstruction will have poor air exchange. The signs of a severe airway obstruction include the following:

- Increased breathing difficulty
- Weak and ineffective cough
- Inability to speak or breathe
- Blue-gray skin, fingernail beds, and inside of the mouth

The person who is choking may also appear panicky and desperate and clutch at his or her throat to communicate that he or she is choking. This motion is known as the universal distress signal for choking.

Caring for Airway Obstruction

For a responsive adult or child with a severe airway obstruction, ask the person, "Are you choking?" If the person is unable to verbally respond but nods yes, provide care for the person. Move behind the person and reach around his or her waist with both arms. Place a fist with the thumb side against the person's abdomen, just above the navel. Grasp the fist with your other hand and press into the abdomen with quick inward and upward thrusts (also known as the Heimlich maneuver). Continue thrusts until the object is removed or the person becomes unresponsive. If your arms cannot encircle the person (eg, woman in last stages of pregnancy, person with obesity), use chest thrusts.

For a responsive infant with a severe airway obstruction, give back blows and chest compressions instead of abdominal thrusts to relieve the obstruction. Support the infant's head and neck and lay the infant facedown on your forearm, then lower your arm to your leg. Give five back blows between the infant's shoulder blades with the heel of your hand. While supporting the back of the infant's head, roll the infant faceup and give five chest compressions with two fingers on the infant's sternum in the same location used for CPR. These are separate and distinct thrusts and are not like the faster CPR compressions. Repeat these steps until the object is removed or the infant becomes unresponsive.

To relieve an airway obstruction in an adult or child, follow the steps in Skill Sheet 6-4. For an infant with an airway obstruction, follow the steps in Skill Sheet 6-5.

Skill Sheet

6-4 Adult and Child Choking

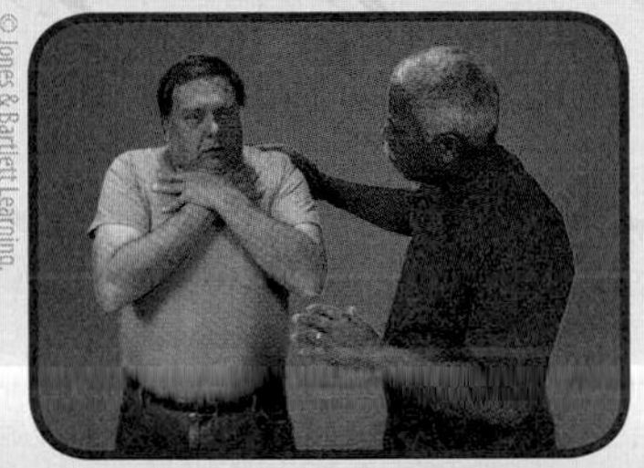

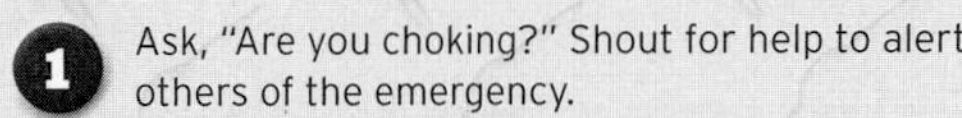

1. Ask, "Are you choking?" Shout for help to alert others of the emergency.

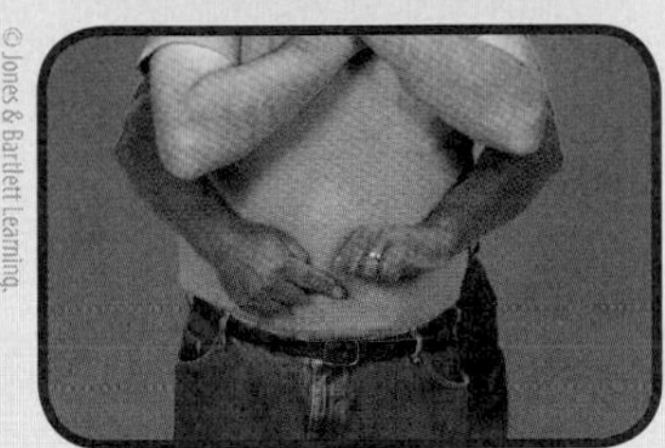

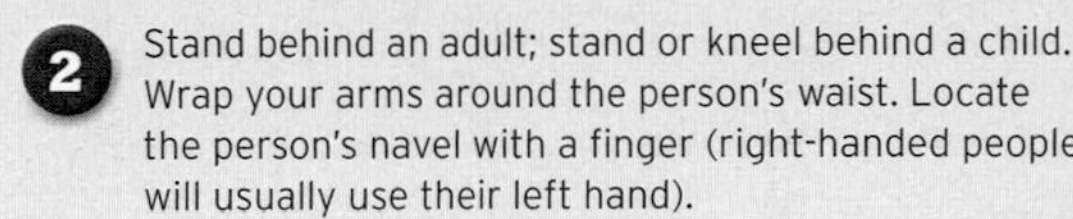

2. Stand behind an adult; stand or kneel behind a child. Wrap your arms around the person's waist. Locate the person's navel with a finger (right-handed people will usually use their left hand).

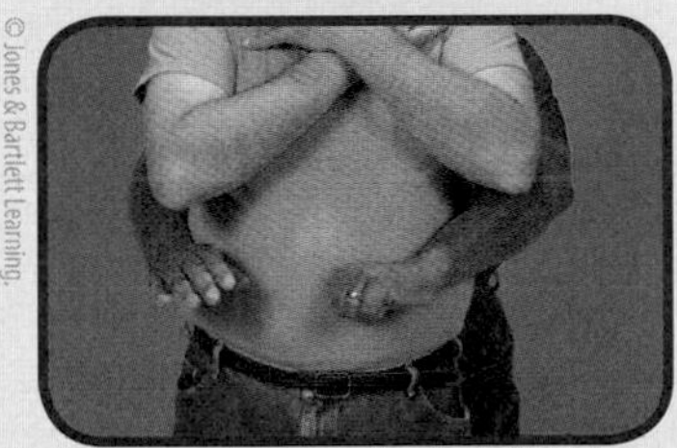

3. Make a fist with the other hand (right-handed people will usually use their right hand) and place the thumb side of the hand just above the person's navel and below the tip of the breast bone.

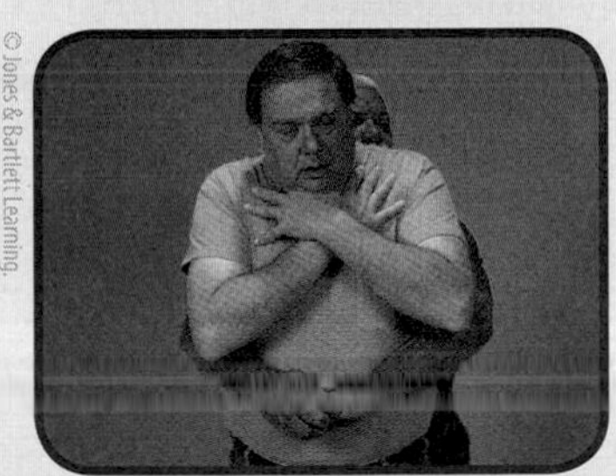

4. Grasp the fist with the other hand. Thrust the fist into the person's abdomen with a quick upward motion. (Use chest thrusts on a person who is choking and obese or pregnant.) Each thrust should be a separate and distinct effort to dislodge the object. Continue without interruption until the person coughs up the object, speaks, moves, or breathes, or EMS or a person who is trained takes over.

5. If the person becomes unresponsive or a person is found unresponsive, provide CPR with the addition of a step:
   - Give 30 chest compressions.
   - Give 2 breaths. If the first breath does not cause the chest to rise, retilt the head and attempt a second breath.
   - Continue sets of 30 chest compressions and 2 breaths. Each time before giving the first of the 2 breaths, look into the mouth for an object; if seen, remove it.

Skill Sheet

6-5 Infant Choking

Note: An infant is not breathing if he or she is unable to cry or make a sound.

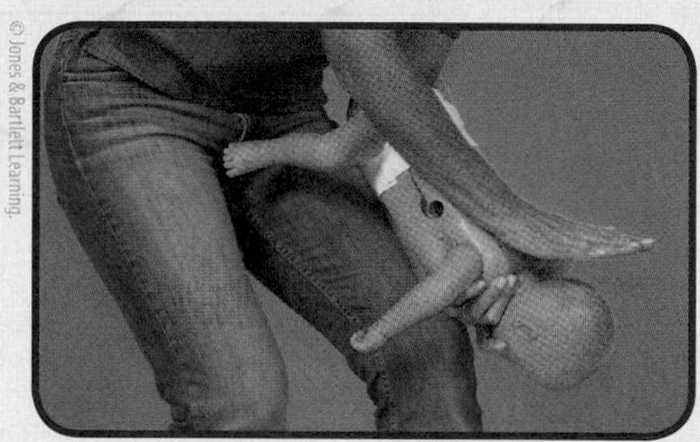

1. Give up to 5 separate and distinct back blows.
   - Support the infant's head with your hand.
   - Lay the infant facedown over your forearm, with the head lower than his or her chest.
   - Brace your forearm and the infant against your thigh.
   - Give the back blows between the infant's shoulder blades with the heel of your other hand.
   - If the object does not come out, turn the infant onto his or her back while supporting the head.

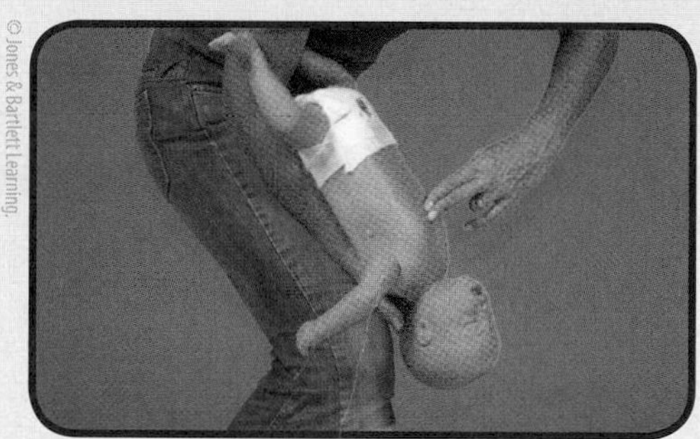

2. Give up to 5 separate and distinct chest thrusts.
   - Support the infant's head with your hand.
   - Lay the infant faceup over your forearm, with the head lower than his or her chest.
   - Brace your forearm and the infant against your thigh.
   - Place 2 fingers of your other hand in same location as giving CPR compressions.
   - Give the thrusts 1 sec apart—this is not as fast as CPR compressions.

3. Continue alternating the 5 back blows and 5 chest thrusts without interruption until the infant stops responding or can breathe, cough, or cry, or until EMS or a person who is trained takes over.

4. If the infant is found or becomes unresponsive:
   - Give 30 chest compressions.
   - Look into the infant's mouth for an object; if seen, remove it.
   - Give 2 breaths.

▶ Automated External Defibrillator

An AED is an electronic device that analyzes the heart rhythm and if necessary delivers an electric shock, known as defibrillation, to the heart of a person in cardiac arrest. The purpose of this shock is to correct an abnormal electrical disturbance and reestablish a heart rhythm that will result in normal electrical and pumping function.

The AED is attached to a cable that is connected to two adhesive pads (electrodes) that are placed on the person's chest. The pad and cable system sends the electrical signal from the heart into the device for rhythm analysis and delivers the electric shock to the person when needed. This system enables first aid providers and other rescuers to deliver early defibrillation with only minimal training.

Common Elements of AEDs

Many different AED models exist. The principles for use are the same for each, but the displays, controls, and options vary slightly. You will need to know how to use your specific AED.

Using an AED

Follow the sequence in **Skill Sheet 6-6** when it is determined that an AED is needed.

1. Some AEDs power on by pressing an on/off button. Others power on when the AED case lid is opened. Once the power is on, the AED will quickly go through some internal checks and will then begin to provide voice and screen prompts.
2. Expose the person's chest. The skin must be fairly dry so that the pads will adhere and conduct electricity properly. If necessary, dry the skin with a towel. Because excessive chest hair may also interfere with adhesion and electrical conduction, you may need to quickly shave the area where the pads are to be placed.
3. Remove the backing from the pads and apply them firmly to the person's bare chest according to the diagram on the pads. One pad is placed to the right of the breast bone, just below the collar bone and above the right nipple. The second pad is placed on the left side of the chest, left of the nipple and above the lower rib margin.
4. Make sure the cable is attached to the AED, and stand clear for analysis of the heart's electrical activity. No one should be in contact with the person at this time, or later if a shock is indicated.
5. Verify that no one is in contact with the person. The AED will advise of the need to shock and, depending on the device, either will advise you to push a button to administer the shock or will deliver the shock automatically. Begin CPR immediately following the shock, and follow the prompts, which will include

reanalyzing the heart rhythm (about every five sets of CPR). If the shock worked, the person will begin to move. Continue providing care until EMS arrives and takes over.

DO NOT use the AED in water. Because water conducts electricity, the electrical current may move across the person's skin rather than between the pads to the person's heart. If the person is submerged in water, then pull him or her out of the water and quickly wipe off as much moisture as possible from the chest before attaching the AED pads.

Skill Sheet

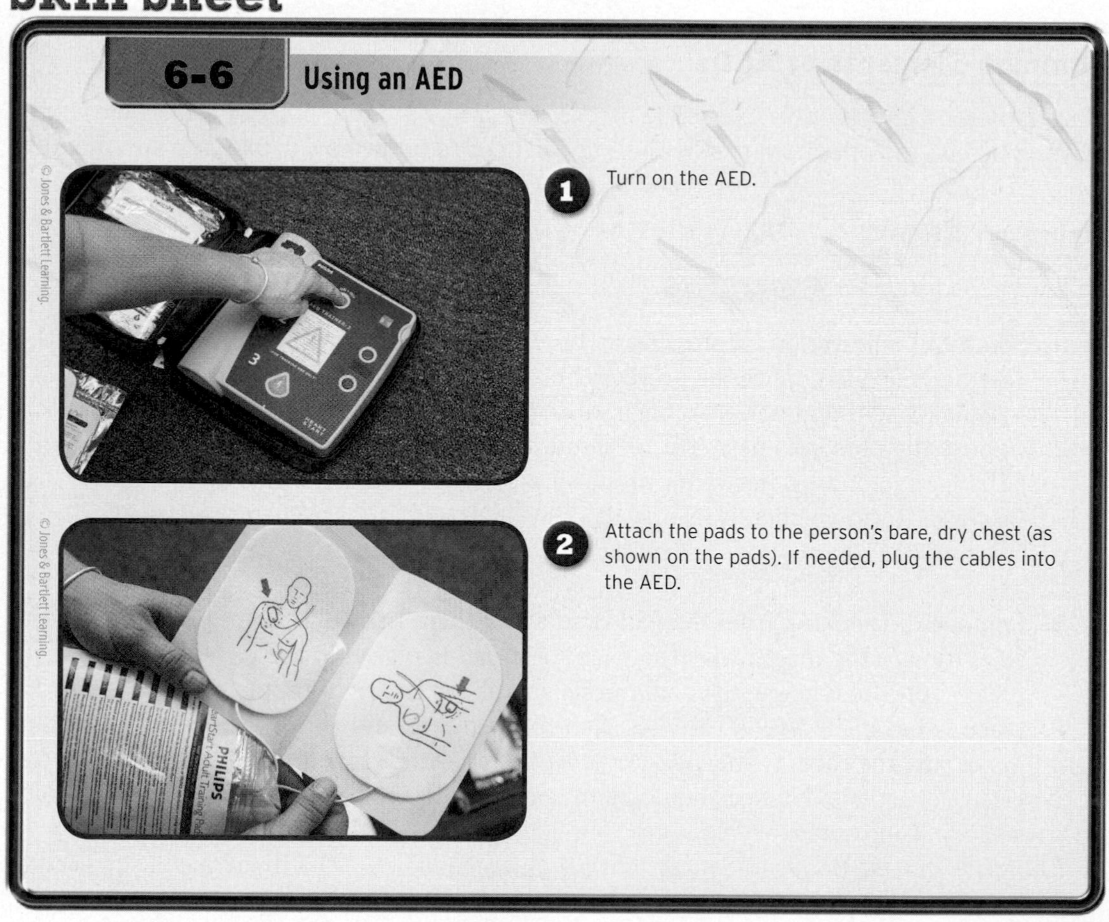

6-6 Using an AED

1. Turn on the AED.
2. Attach the pads to the person's bare, dry chest (as shown on the pads). If needed, plug the cables into the AED.

Skill Sheet Continued

6-6 Using an AED

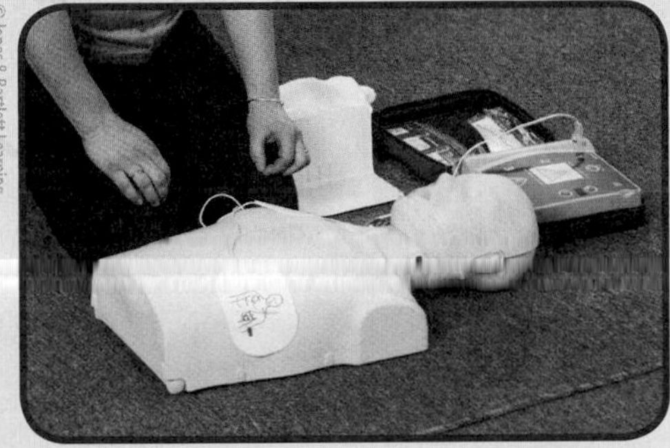

© Jones & Bartlett Learning.

3 Stay clear of the person. Make sure no one, including you, is touching the person. Say, "Clear!"

Allow the AED to analyze the heart rhythm (push the Analyze button, if necessary).

The AED will prompt one of three actions:

- Press shock button.
- Stay clear while the AED automatically delivers a shock.
- Do not shock but give CPR, starting with chest compressions with the pads staying in place.

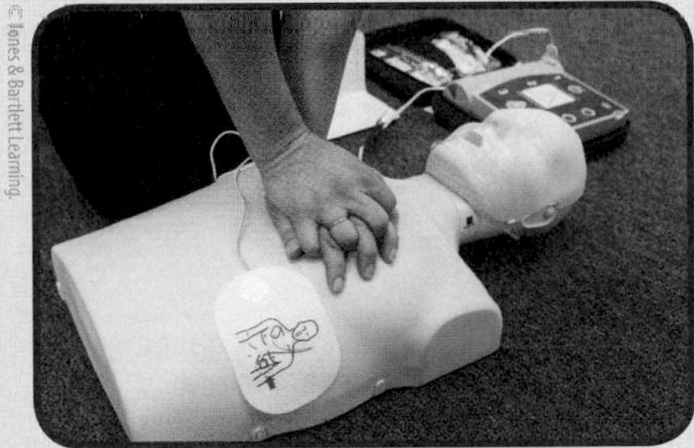

© Jones & Bartlett Learning.

4 After any one of the three actions, give 5 sets of CPR unless the person moves, begins to breathe, or wakes up.

5 Repeat Steps 3 and 4 until the person moves or begins to breathe, or until EMS takes over.

Quick Review of CPR and AED Procedures Using the RAB-CAB Procedure

Steps/Action	Adults (at or past puberty)	Child (1 year to puberty)	Infant (younger than 1 year)
R = Responsive?			
Technique	Tap a shoulder and shout, "Are you OK?" A person who is responsive will answer, move, or moan.		Tap the bottom of a foot and shout his or her name. A responsive infant will cry or move.
A = Activate EMS and get an AED. (Shout for nearby help and call 9-1-1 or the emergency response number. An AED may or may not be available.)			
When?	• If you are alone, call 9-1-1 and get an AED. When you return, use the AED. • If another person is with you, send him or her to call and get an AED while you begin CPR immediately.	• If you are alone, and before calling 9-1-1, give 5 sets of 30 chest compressions and 2 breaths (CPR). • After 5 sets of CPR, leave the child or infant to call 9-1-1 and get an AED. • When you return, use the AED on the child as soon as possible.	
Whom to call?	Call 9-1-1 or the emergency response number.		
B = Breathing? Check for no breathing or only gasping.			
• Place person faceup on a flat, firm surface. • Observe the face and chest movement for breathing. Take 5 sec but no more than 10 sec.	If the person is not breathing or is only occasionally gasping (may sound like a quick inhalation or like a groan/snore), CPR is needed. If the person is breathing but not responding, CPR is not needed; place the person in the recovery position to keep his or her airway clear, and monitor breathing.		
C = Chest compressions			
Where to place person?	Firm, flat surface (eg, floor, ground, sidewalk)		Can be placed on table or cabinet top
Where to place hands?	Center of chest and lower half of breast bone (sternum)		Pads of 2 fingers in the center of chest on the breast bone with 1 touching and both below the imaginary nipple line
	2 hands: • Heel of 1 hand on breast bone; other hand on top • Fingers of both hands interlocked • Arms straight with shoulders directly over the hands	1 hand for very small child: Heel of 1 hand only 2 hands: • Same as for an adult • Arms straight with shoulders directly over the hands	

Quick Review of CPR and AED Procedures Using the RAB-CAB Procedure

<table>
<tr><th>Steps/Action</th><th>Adults (at or past puberty)</th><th>Child (1 year to puberty)</th><th>Infant (younger than 1 year)</th></tr>
<tr><td rowspan="2">Depth</td><td>At least 2 in. (5 cm) but no more than 2.4 in. (6 cm)</td><td>About 2 in. (5 cm) or at least 1/3 depth of the upper body (chest)</td><td>About 1.5 in. (4 cm) or at least 1/3 depth of the upper body (chest)</td></tr>
<tr><td colspan="3">After each compression, allow full recoil of the chest.
DO NOT lean on the chest of an adult or child.</td></tr>
<tr><td>Rate</td><td colspan="3">100–120 per min
(Follow the beat of the Bee Gees song "Stayin' Alive," the beats from a smartphone application that was previously installed and is quickly accessible, or a dispatcher's directions heard over a cell phone's speaker.)</td></tr>
<tr><td>Ratio of chest compressions to breaths</td><td colspan="3">30:2</td></tr>
<tr><td colspan="4">**A = Airway open**</td></tr>
<tr><td>Technique</td><td colspan="3">Head tilt-chin lift</td></tr>
<tr><td colspan="4">**B = Breaths**</td></tr>
<tr><td rowspan="2">Technique</td><td colspan="2">• Pinch the nose shut, and, with your mouth, make an airtight mouth-to-mouth seal. Use a CPR mask or face shield, if available.
• Perform the head tilt-chin lift maneuver.
• Give 2 breaths:
  • Each breath should last 1 sec.
  • Blow enough to make the chest rise.</td><td rowspan="2">Perform the head tilt-chin lift maneuver (do not tilt the head back too far).
• Cover the infant's mouth and nose with your mouth, making an airtight seal. If this does not work, try either mouth-to-mouth or mouth-to-nose breaths.
• Give 2 breaths:
  • Each breath should last 1 sec.
  • Blow enough to make the chest rise.</td></tr>
<tr><td colspan="2">If first breath does not cause chest to rise, retilt head and give second breath. If second breath does not make chest rise, begin CPR (30 compressions and 2 breaths). Each time before giving a breath, open the mouth and look for an object; if seen, remove it.</td></tr>
<tr><td colspan="4">Continue CPR until:
1. The person begins breathing.
2. Other rescuer(s) (ie, trained layperson, EMS personnel) take over.</td></tr>
</table>

(*continues*)

Quick Review of CPR and AED Procedures Using the RAB-CAB Procedure

Steps/Action	Adults (at or past puberty)	Child (1 year to puberty)	Infant (younger than 1 year)

3. An AED arrives and is used (except for infants).
4. You become physically exhausted and unable to continue.

If another person is available, trade off about every 5 sets of CPR (2 min).

Defibrillation

If available, use an AED as soon as possible.

1. Turn on the AED.
2. Attach the pads on the person's bare, dry chest (shown on the pads' diagrams). If needed, plug the cables into the AED. Child-sized pads may be available.
3. Stay clear of the person. Make sure no one, including you, is touching the person. Say, "Clear!"
4. Allow the AED to analyze the heart rhythm (push Analyze button, if necessary). The AED will prompt one of three actions:
   - Stay clear while the AED automatically delivers a shock.
   - Press the shock button.
   - Do not shock but give CPR, starting with chest compressions with the pads staying in place.

After performing any one of the three actions, give 5 sets of CPR unless the person moves, begins to breathe, or wakes up.

Repeat defibrillation Steps 2 and 3 until the person moves, begins to breathe, or wakes up, or EMS arrives and takes over.

© Boston Globe/Getty.

7 Emergency Rescues, Moves, and Priorities

Chapter at a glance

▶ Emergency Rescues

Before attempting an emergency rescue, size up the scene (see page 8).

- Are dangerous hazards present?
- How many people are involved?
- What happened?
- Are bystanders available to help?

If the scene is dangerous, **DO NOT** attempt to rescue. Call 9-1-1. Several types of rescues require special training and equipment.

What to Look For	What to Do
Water	Try the following methods in the order listed: 1. Reach the person from shore with a pole, long stick, or other similar object. 2. Throw anything that floats (eg, empty picnic jug, piece of wood) to the person. 3. Row to the person, if a boat is available. Wear a personal flotation device. 4. Go to the person, if you are a capable swimmer trained in water lifesaving procedures. Use a towel or board for the person to grab. **DO NOT** let the person grab you.
Ice	1. If near the shore, reach the person with a pole or throw a line with an object that floats attached. 2. If unsuccessful, lie flat on the ice and push a ladder, plank, or similar object ahead of you.
Electricity	1. High-voltage electricity requires trained personnel. 2. If indoors, turn off the electricity.
Motor-vehicle crash	1. Park in a safe place. 2. Turn on flashers. 3. Place flares or reflectors 250 to 500 feet (75 to 150 m) behind the crash.
Fire	1. Get people out of the area. 2. If it is a small fire, use a fire extinguisher if you can easily escape.
Hazardous materials	1. Stay out of the area. 2. If outside, stay upwind.
Confined space (an area lacking fresh air; toxic vapors may be present)	Only those with proper training and equipment should enter the area.

Emergency Moves

As a first aid provider, you will seldom need to move an injured person because most injured people can do so by themselves. For severe injuries, waiting for emergency medical services (EMS) to arrive is often the best decision. Only move a person if immediate danger exists Table 7-1, such as the following:

- A fire or danger of a fire
- Involvement of explosives or other hazardous materials

Table 7-1 Emergency Rescue Moves

Moves for Two First Aid Providers	When to Use
Two-person assist Figure 7-1	Used when person has a leg injury
Two-handed seat carry Figure 7-2	Used when no equipment is available and the person cannot walk but can use the arms to hang onto the two first aid providers
Extremity carry Figure 7-3	Used when no equipment is available and the person cannot walk and cannot use the arms to hang onto the two first aid providers
Chair carry Figure 7-4	Used for narrow passage or up or down stairs when a chair is available
Moves for One First Aid Provider	**When to Use**
Human crutch Figure 7-5	Used when person has a leg injury
Cradle carry Figure 7-6	Used for children and lightweight adults who cannot walk
Pack-strap carry Figure 7-7	Used for long distances when injuries make carrying the person over the first aid provider's shoulder unsafe
Piggyback carry Figure 7-8	Used when the person cannot walk but can use the arms to hang onto the first aid provider
Firefighter's carry Figure 7-9	Used for long distances when the person can be carried over the first aid provider's shoulder
Shoulder drag Figure 7-10	Used for short distances over a rough surface
Ankle drag Figure 7-11	Used for short distances over a smooth surface
Blanket drag Figure 7-12	Used for short distances

- Inability to protect the scene from hazards
- Inability to gain access to other persons who need lifesaving care (eg, vehicle crash)

You may also encounter situations in which you must move a person to provide first aid Flowchart 7-1, such as the following:

- Giving cardiopulmonary resuscitation (CPR) that requires a firm, flat surface
- Placing an unresponsive, breathing person in the recovery position
- Positioning a person to treat for shock

Cautions about moving a person include the following:

- **DO NOT** move a person unless absolutely necessary (ie, the person is in immediate danger or must be moved to shelter while waiting for EMS to arrive).

- **DO NOT** make an injury worse by moving the person.
- **DO NOT** move a person who could have a spinal injury unless it is absolutely necessary due to other threats to life, such as a fire or threat of a fire, hazardous materials, or explosives.
- **DO NOT** move a person unless you know where you are going.
- **DO NOT** move a person without stabilizing the injured part.
- **DO NOT** move a person when you can send someone for help. Wait with the person.
- **DO NOT** try to move a person by yourself if other people are available to help.
- **DO NOT** enter certain hazardous areas (eg, a confined space filled with a gas or vapors) unless you have the proper training and equipment.

When lifting a person, use proper techniques to protect yourself against injury:

- Know your capabilities. **DO NOT** try to handle a load that is too heavy or awkward; seek help.
- Use a safe grip. Use as much of your palms as possible.
- Bend your knees to use the strong muscles of the thighs and buttocks.
- Keep your arms close to your body and your elbows flexed.
- Position your feet shoulder width apart for balance, one in front of the other.

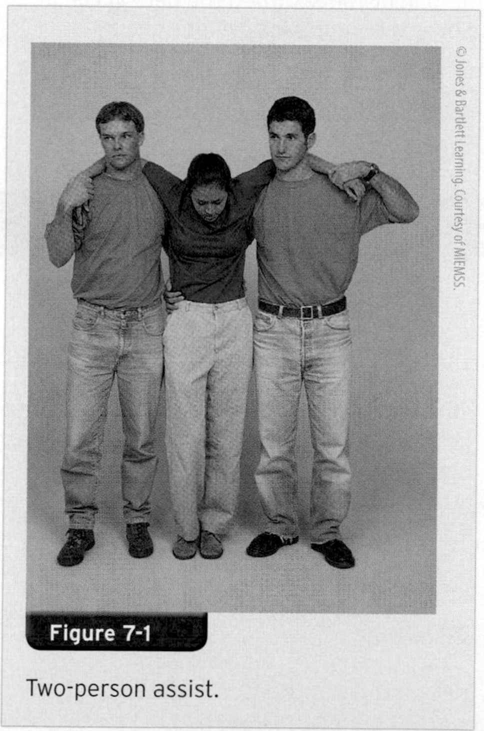

Figure 7-1

Two-person assist.

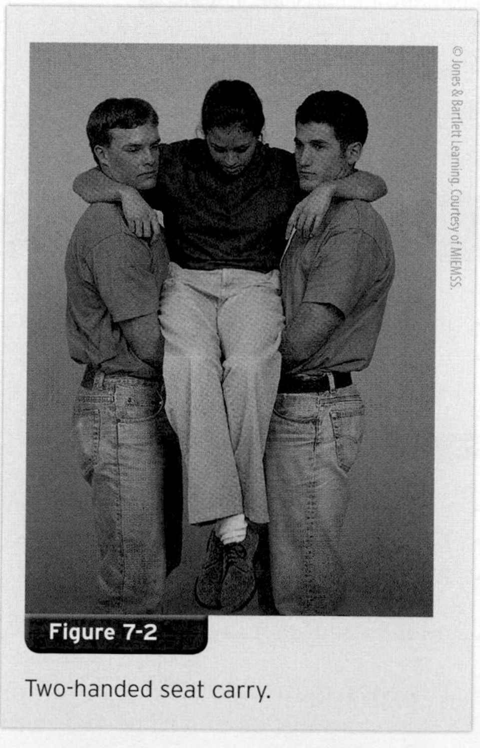

Figure 7-2

Two-handed seat carry.

- When lifting, keep and lift the person close to your body.
- While lifting, **DO NOT** twist your back; pivot with your feet.
- Lift and carry slowly, smoothly, and in unison with the other lifter.
- Before you move a person, explain to him or her what you are doing.

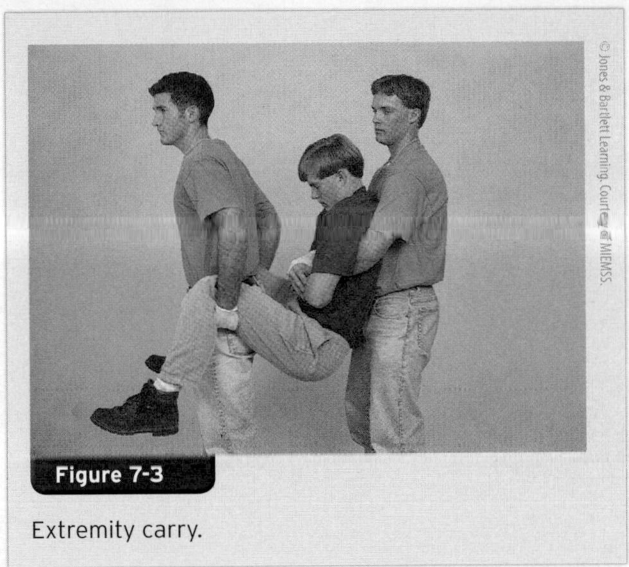

Figure 7-3

Extremity carry.

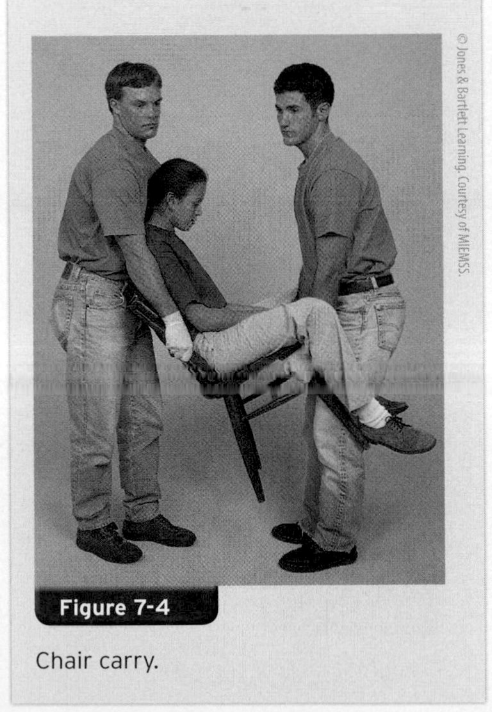

Figure 7-4

Chair carry.

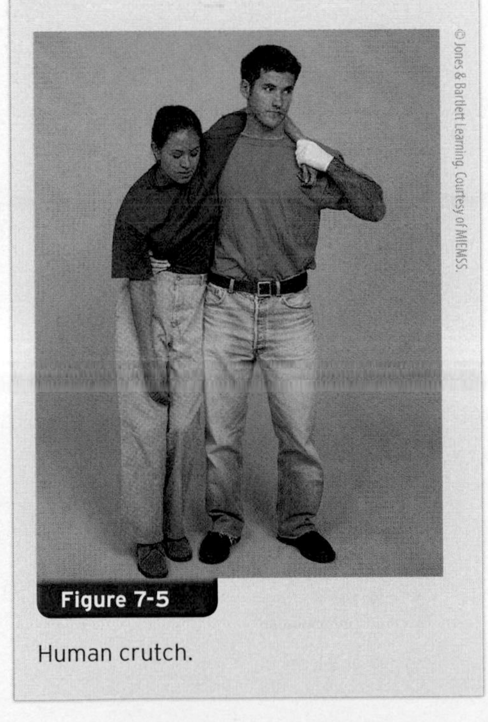

Figure 7-5

Human crutch.

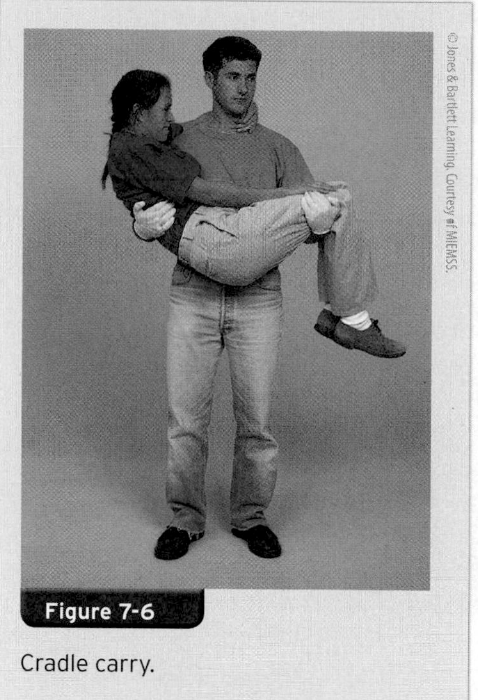

Figure 7-6

Cradle carry.

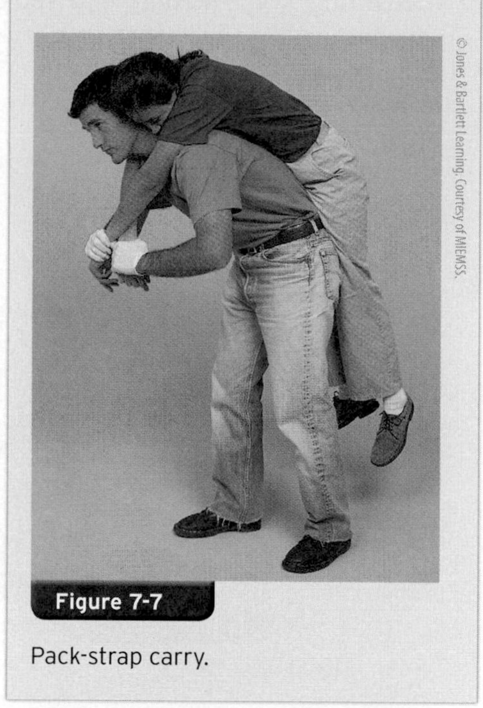

Figure 7-7

Pack-strap carry.

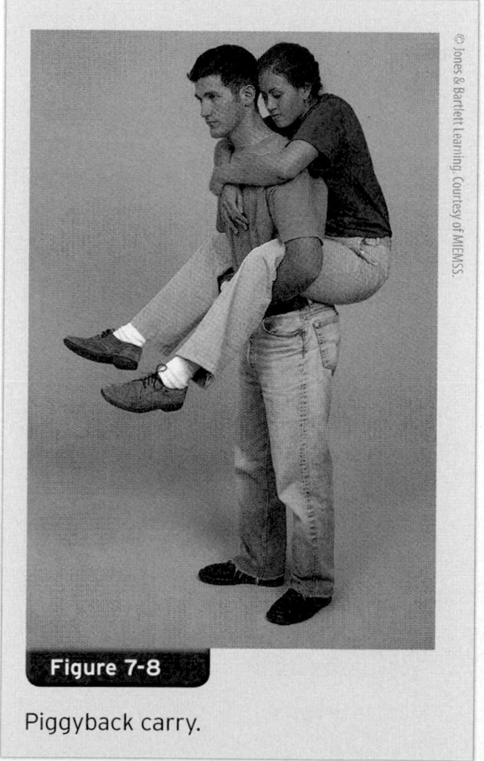

Figure 7-8

Piggyback carry.

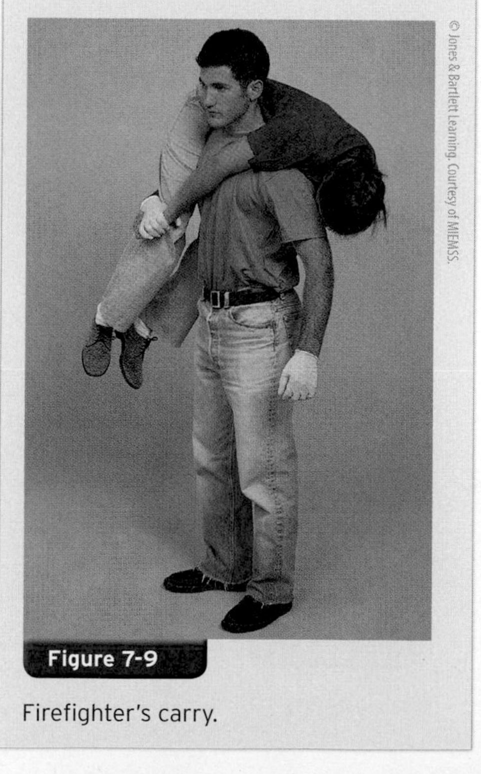

Figure 7-9

Firefighter's carry.

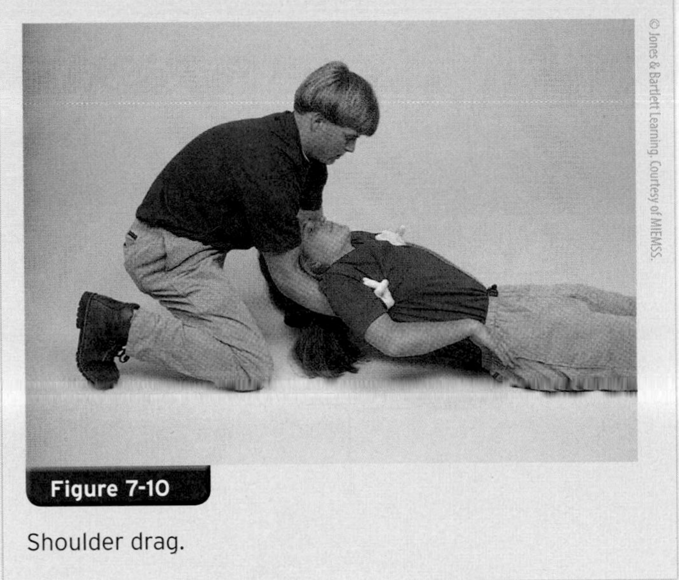

Figure 7-10

Shoulder drag.

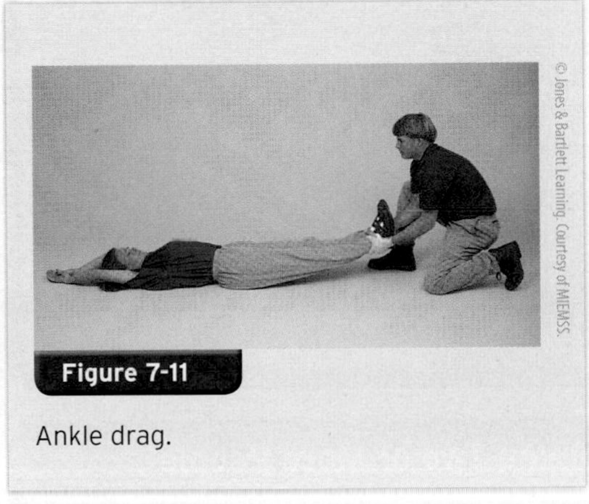

Figure 7-11

Ankle drag.

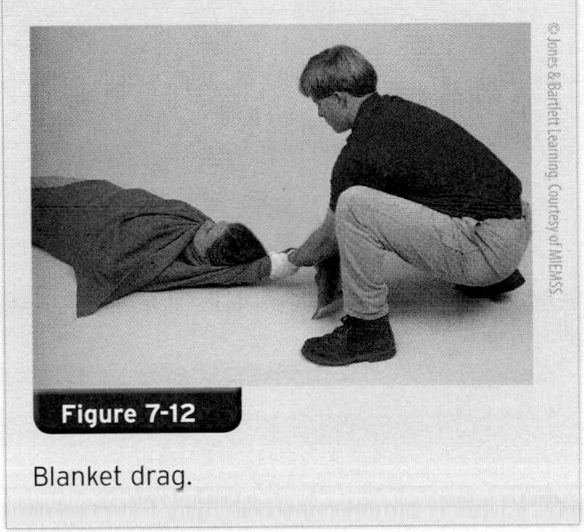

Figure 7-12

Blanket drag.

▶ Prioritizing Multiple Injured People

Situations requiring first aid usually involve only one person. Rarely will you encounter a large-scale event involving more than one person needing care. Such events may seem commonplace because when they do occur, they are frequently reported in the mass media **Table 7-2**.

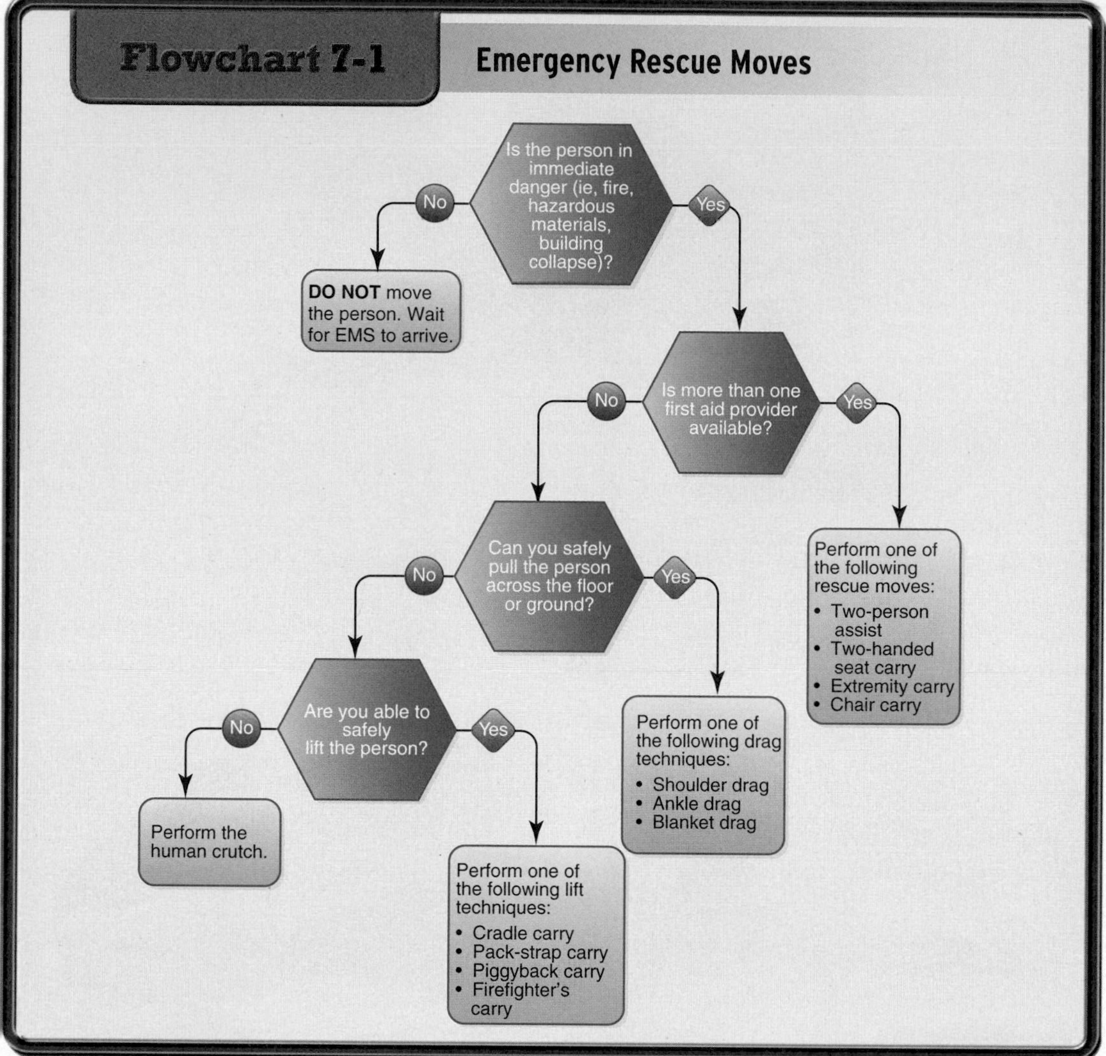

Table 7-2 Examples of Disasters Involving Two or More People

Natural Disasters	Human-Caused Disasters
Earthquakes	Highway crashes
Tornadoes	Air crashes
Hurricanes	Train derailments
Floods	Terrorist attacks
Lightning strikes	Mass shootings
Heat waves	Explosions

When many people are injured, use a process called triage (a French word meaning "to sort") to distinguish among:

- Those needing immediate care for one of the three "killers"—closed airway, severe bleeding, and shock
- Those who can wait for care until after others have been triaged
- Those who are deceased (dead)

Triage's intent is to provide the greatest good for the greatest number of people. Some people have a greater need for emergency care than others. Someone has to go last.

Triage is especially effective in situations in which:

- There are more injured people than first aid providers and rescuers.
- Time is critical.

Triage Categories

During triage, you should evaluate and sort every injured person into one of three categories Table 7-3.

While EMS personnel may have ribbons, cards, or tags to place on people to identify their category, you will rarely have these items. You can, however, improvise (eg, write on a piece of tape placed on the person's forehead or around the wrist). After triage, take the injured, according to their category, to a medical facility, if available, or to an area designated for medical treatment.

Conducting Triage

Step 1: Conduct a voice triage by calling out, "If you can walk, come to me." People who can get up and walk rarely have life-threatening injuries. Do not force a person to move if he or she complains of pain. People who can walk can be placed in the "delayed" category. Direct them to a designated safe area; have them sit down and stay together. If you need more assistance, you can ask for volunteers from this group to help.

Table 7-3 Triage Categories

Category	Description
Immediate	Person has life-threatening injuries (airway closed, severe bleeding, or shock) demanding immediate action to save his or her life.
Delayed	Person's life is not threatened. He or she may need care, but it can be delayed while other people are triaged.
Dead/deceased	Person is not breathing after his or her airway has been opened. There may be no time or people to do CPR when others need immediate help. A volunteer from the "walking wounded" group might be able to perform compression-only CPR or, if trained, CPR. An exception to "bypassing the dead" to treat the moderately or severely injured occurs when a lightning strike involves multiple people; in this event, CPR should be given to those motionless but appearing to be dead before aiding people in other categories.

Step 2: Start surveying each person who did not get up and walk. Begin with the person closest to where you are standing. Quickly get to each person and sort each by his or her need for care. Tag everyone as "immediate," "delayed," or "dead." **DO NOT** stop to treat anyone during triage except to quickly open the airway and control severe bleeding.

When performing triage Flowchart 7-2:

- If a person fails one of the tests (or checks), tag him or her as "immediate."
- If a person passes all of the tests (or checks), tag as "delayed."
- Everyone should get a tag.

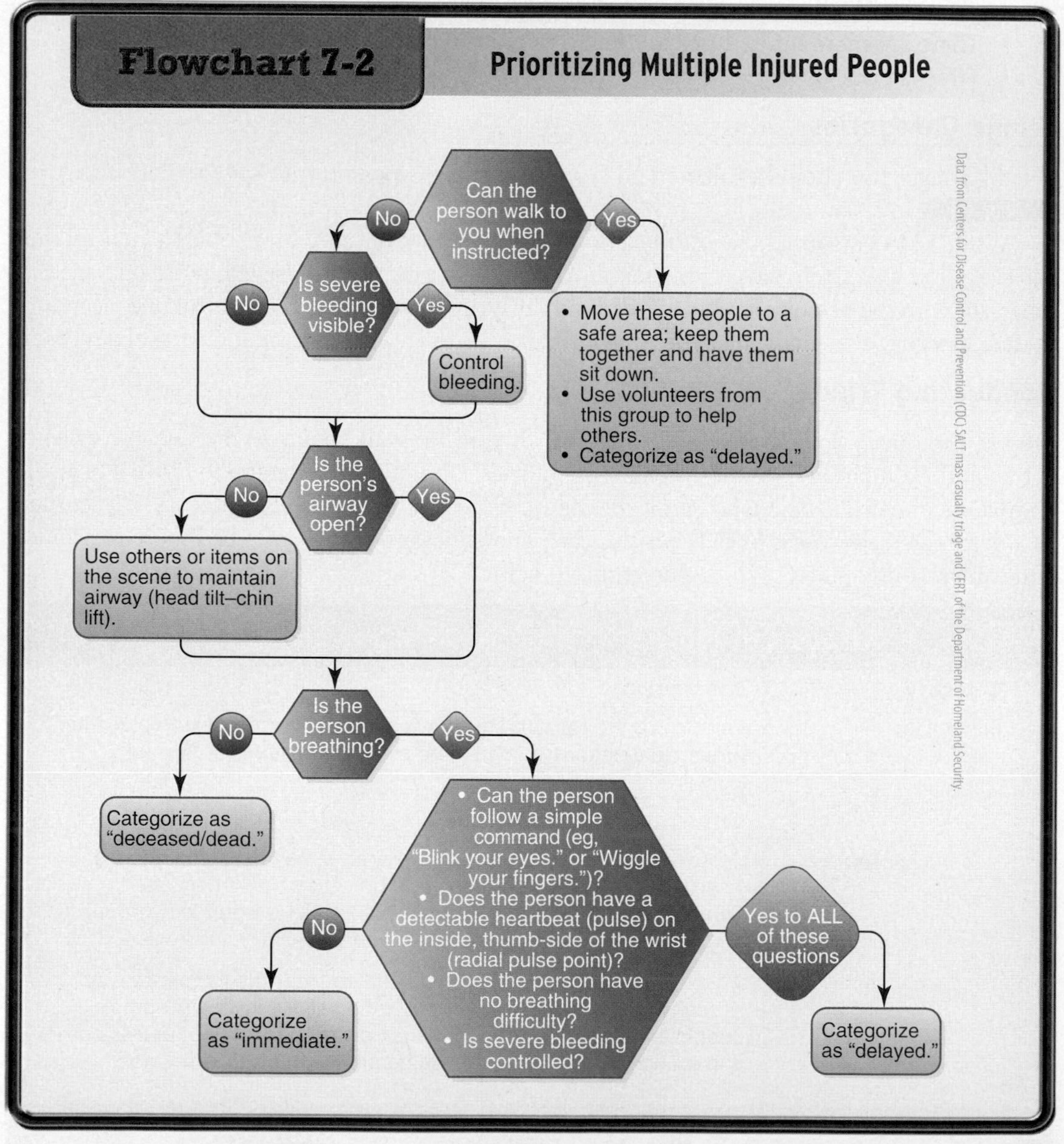

First Aid Supplies

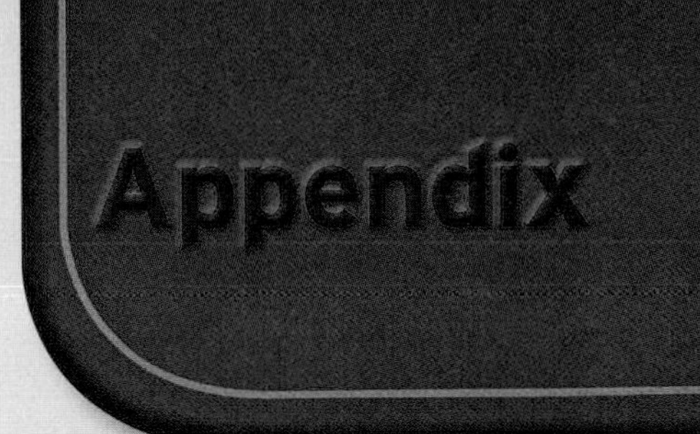

▶ First Aid Supplies

Supplies in a first aid kit should be customized to include those items that are likely to be used, including nonprescription (over-the-counter [OTC]) medications. Some medications lose their potency over time, especially after they have been opened; check expiration dates twice a year. Keep all medications out of the reach of children and use child-resistant containers. Read and follow all directions for proper medication use. For first aid kits for workplaces, schools, and public places, do not include products known to cause drowsiness (eg, antihistamine).

The perfect first aid kit does not exist; include items for injuries and sudden illnesses you are likely to encounter Table A-1. Do not fill a first aid kit with items you do not know how to use.

Table A-1 Sample Items for a First Aid Kit

Items for Bleeding Control	
Disposable medical exam gloves (non-latex)	Protects against potentially infected blood, body fluids, or contaminated items
Hemostatic wound dressing	Use only when direct pressure fails to control bleeding.
Tourniquet	Use only when direct pressure fails to control bleeding.
Items for Wound Care	
Alcohol hand sanitizer (small bottle)	Cleans hands and the area around the wound (not inside wound)
Antibiotic ointment (Polysporin, Neosporin, Bacitracinor triple-antibiotic ointment)	Prevents skin infections that are associated with shallow wounds and helps to prevent dressings from sticking to the wound
Surgical tape (Micropore paper tape) (1 in. and 2 in. [3 cm and 5 cm])	Covers blisters
Elastic tape (Elastikon) (2 in. and 4 in. [5 cm and 10 cm])	Covers wounds and blisters
Blister pad (Spenco 2nd Skin) (1 in. and 3 in. [3 cm and 7 cm])	Covers wounds and blisters
Adhesive bandage strips (1 in. × 3 in. [3 cm × 7 cm] and other various sizes)	Covers minor wounds

(continues)

Table A-1 Sample Items for a First Aid Kit (continued)

Sterile gauze pads (3 in. × 3 in. and 4 in. × 4 in. [7 cm × 7 cm and 10 cm × 10 cm]; individually wrapped)	Covers wounds
Nonstick pads (3 in. × 4 in. [7 cm × 10 cm])	Covers burns, blisters, and scrapes
Self-adhering roller gauze bandage (2 in., 3 in., and 4 in. [5 cm, 7 cm, and 10 cm] wide)	Holds dressings in place
Sterile trauma pad (5 in. × 9 in., 8 in. × 10 in. [13 cm × 23 cm, 20 cm × 25 cm])	Covers large wounds
Triangular bandage (40 in. × 40 in. × 56 in. [102 cm × 102 cm × 142 cm])	Two triangular bandages can make an arm sling and a binder. When folded, it can hold dressings and splints in place.
Sterile eye pads	Cover both eyes to prevent both eyes from moving, even if only one is injured.
Items for Bone, Joint, and Muscle Care	
Cold pack (instant and disposable)	Use on sprains, dislocations, fractures, and insect stings when ice is not available.
Splint (padded and malleable, such as a SAM Splint)	Stabilizes broken bones and dislocations
Elastic bandage (3 in. [7 cm] wide)	Provides compression to reduce the swelling of joint injuries
Plastic bags (sealable)	Holds ice to apply on insect stings and bone, joint, and muscle injuries; contains embedded tick after its removal
Nonprescription (OTC) Medications *Keep all medications out of the reach of children and use child-resistant containers. For schools and worksites, giving oral medications is often prohibited; check the policies.*	
Glucose tablets	Treats hypoglycemia (low blood sugar)
Acetaminophen (Tylenol)	Treats pain and fever
Ibuprofen (Advil)	Treats pain, fever, and inflammation
Aspirin (Motrin)	Treats pain, fever, and inflammation; may be used for suspected heart attack. **DO NOT** give aspirin to children.
Antihistamine (Benadryl) *Warning*: First aid kits at workplaces, schools, and public places should not contain products known to cause drowsiness.	Relieves allergy symptoms; treats poison ivy or oak itching and rash; reduces nausea and motion sickness; causes drowsiness and induces sleep
Hydrocortisone cream, 1%	Relieves itchiness and skin-related reactions, including rashes associated with insect bites and stings, poison ivy and oak, and other allergic skin rashes. It may be too weak for some conditions.

(*continues*)

Table A-1 Sample Items for a First Aid Kit (continued)

Aloe vera gel (100% gel)	Treats sunburn or superficial frostbite
Sports drink packets (eg, Gatorade, Powerade)	Treats heat stress, dehydration, and water intoxication when too much water has been consumed and sodium has been depleted from the body
Antacids tablets (eg, Tums and Rolaids)	Treats heartburn and acid indigestion (upset stomach)
Antidiarrheal tablets (eg, Pepto-Bismol and Imodium A-D)	Treats diarrhea
Anticonstipation/laxative tablets (eg, Metamucil)	Treats constipation
Equipment	
Cardiopulmonary resuscitation (CPR) breathing barrier device (with 1-way valve)	Protects against potential infection during CPR
Scissors (various types available)	Cuts dressings, bandages, and clothing
Tweezers (angled tip)	Removes splinters and ticks
Safety pins (2 in. [5 cm] long)	Creates sling from shirttail or sleeve, secures dressings, and drains blisters
Emergency blanket (eg, large household polyethylene trash bags, space blanket made of Mylar, although it may tear in wind)	Protects against body heat loss and weather (wind, rain, and snow)
First Aid and CPR Guide (first aid booklet from Jones & Bartlett Learning)	Provides quick reference during an emergency and for review of first aid procedures

Workplace First Aid Kit Contents

In the absence of a medical facility in close proximity to a workplace, the Occupational Safety and Health Administration (OSHA) requires that the workplace have adequate supplies readily available and a person or people at the workplace who are adequately trained to render first aid to all injured employees. Neither OSHA's general industry standard 1910.151 nor its construction standard 1926.50 require specific contents be included in the workplace first aid kit.

OSHA refers to the American National Standard (ANSI) z308.1, *Minimum Requirements for Workplace First Aid Kits*, for minimum items to include in a workplace first aid kit. These items, as well as other recommended supplies, are included in Table A-2.

Table A-2 Recommended Minimum Items for a Workplace First Aid Kit

Equipment	Minimum Quantity
Adhesive bandage (1 in. × 3 in. [3 cm × 7 cm])	16
Adhesive tape (1 in. [3 cm] width)	1 roll
Antibiotic ointment	10 packets
Antiseptic towelette/swab	10 packets
Aspirin (chewable; 81 mg each)	2 packets
Burn dressing (gel soaked; 4 in. × 4 in. [10 cm × 10 cm])	1 packet
Burn treatment	10 packets
Cold pack (instant, disposable)	1
CPR breathing barrier (face mask with 1-way valve)	1
Disposable medical exam gloves (non-latex, large size)	2 pairs
Elastic bandage (3 in. or 4 in. [7 cm or 10 cm] width)	1
Eye covering (0.25 in. [0.64 cm] thick)	2 pads
Eye/skin wash (4-oz [118-mL] bottle)	1 bottle
First Aid and CPR Guide (booklet from Jones & Bartlett Learning)	1
Hand sanitizer (alcohol)	1 small bottle or 10 packets
Roller gauze bandage (3 in. [7 cm] width)	2
Roller gauze bandage (4 in. [10 cm] width)	1
Scissors	1
Splint (malleable, padded such as SAM Splint, 4 in. × 36 in. [10 cm × 91 cm])	1
Sterile gauze pad (3 in. × 3 in. [7 cm × 7 cm])	4, individually wrapped
Sterile trauma pad (5 in. × 9 in. [13 cm × 23 cm])	2, individually wrapped
Tourniquet	1
Triangular bandage (40 in. × 40 in. × 56 in. [102 cm × 102 cm × 142 cm])	2

Note: Nonprescription medications can be put in first aid kits if packaged in single dose, tamper-evident packaging and labeled as required by FDA regulations. OTC drug products should not contain ingredients known to cause drowsiness.

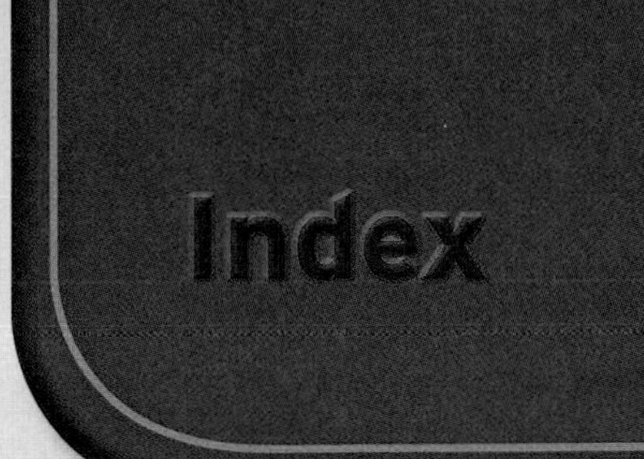

Note: Page numbers followed by *f*, or *t* indicate material in figures, or tables, respectively.

A

B

E

F

R

S

T

U

V

W